The Cleft Palate Story

The Cleft Palate Story

Samuel Berkowitz, DDS, MS, FICD

Orthodontist
Clinical Professor of Pediatrics and Surgery
University of Miami School of Medicine
Research Director, Plastic Surgery Department
Miami Children's Hospital
Miami, Florida

quintessence books

Quintessence Publishing Co, Inc
Chicago, Berlin, London, Tokyo,
São Paulo, Moscow, and Warsaw

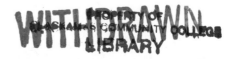

Library of Congress Cataloging-In-Publication Data

Berkowitz, Samuel, 1928-
    The cleft palate story / Samuel Berkowitz.
        p.   cm.
    Includes bibliographical references and index.
    ISBN 0-86715-259-1
        1. Cleft palate—Popular works.   2. Cleft lip—Popular works.
3. Cleft palate children—Rehabilitation.   I. Title.
RD525.B47 1994
617.5'225—dc20   94-7902
                                                                        CIP

© 1994 by Quintessence Publishing Co, Inc

Published by Quintessence Publishing Co, Inc
551 North Kimberly Drive
Carol Stream, IL 60188-1881

Editor: Patricia Bereck Weikersheimer
Design Manager: Jennifer Sabella
Assistant Designer: Lisa Ream

Printed in the United States of America

Contributors

Edward Clifford, PhD
Psychologist
Professor of Medical Psychology
Department of Psychiatry and Department of Surgery
Co-Director of Faculty Rehabilitative Center
Duke University Medical Center
Durham, North Carolina

Sarah Coulter Danner, RN
Pediatric Nurse Practitioner
Affiliated with Monadnock Regional Pediatric Group
Peterborough, New Hampshire

Director, The Lactation Clinic
Cleveland, Ohio

Ronald Haun, MD
Geneticist
Assistant Professor of Clinical Pediatrics and Genetics
University of Miami School of Medicine
Miami, Florida

Leslie M. Holve, MD
Pediatrician
Medical Director
Saint John's Cleft Palate Center
Santa Monica, California
Associate Clinical Professor of Pediatrics
University of California, Los Angeles, School of Medicine
Los Angeles, California

Etoile LeBlanc, MS
Speech/Language Pathologist
Coordinator, Communicative Disorders Program
Center of Craniofacial Disorders
Department of Plastic and Reconstructive Surgery
Montefiore Medical Center
Albert Einstein College of Medicine
Bronx, New York

Linda Linneweh
Coordinator/Administrator, Central Washington Cleft Palate
  Program
Yakima Valley Memorial Hospital
Yakima, Washington

Joan M. McCartney
International Board Certified Lactation Consultant
  and a La Leche Counselor
Sumerville, New Jersey

D. Ralph Millard, Jr, MD, FACS, Hon FRCS Ed
Plastic Surgeon
Light-Millard Professor of Plastic Surgery
Chief of Plastic and Reconstructive Surgery
University of Miami School of Medicine
Director, South Florida Cleft Palate Clinic
Miami, Florida

Robert Shprintzen, PhD
Speech/Language Pathologist
Director, Center for Craniofacial Disorders
Montefiore Medical Center
Professor, Plastic Surgery and Otolaryngology
Albert Einstein College of Medicine
Bronx, New York

Dana K. Smith
Mother of a child with a cleft
White Bear Lake, Minnesota

Sylvan Stool, MD
Otolaryngologist
Director of Education
Department of Otolaryngology
Children's Hospital of Pittsburgh

Professor of Otolaryngology and Pediatrics
University of Pittsburgh School of Medicine
Pittsburgh, Pennsylvania

Mark Webman, DDS
Pediatric Dentist
Chairman, Department of Pediatric Dentistry
Past Chief, Dental Clinic
Miami Children's Hospital
Miami, Florida

S. Anthony Wolfe, MD, FACS
Plastic-Craniofacial Surgeon
Clinical Professor of Plastic and Reconstructive Surgery
University of Miami, School of Medicine

Chief, Division of Plastic Surgery
Miami Children's Hospital
Miami, Florida

To my wife, Lynnie, and my children Beth and Debra.

To the children with facial and palatal clefts, and their parents who have supported my clinical and research efforts, to whom I owe a great deal for allowing me to know and treat them.

Contents

Preface

After more than thirty years of treating children with various types of clefts of the lip and palate and counseling them and their parents, it is clear to me that parents, at the time of the birth of a child with a cleft, need more information on cleft lip and palate than is available from generalized pamphlets. Since the birth of a baby with a cleft lip and/or palate is likely to be unanticipated (the condition usually cannot be detected before birth except by the use of an ultrasound, and then only for some cleft types), the hospital personnel involved in the delivery and nursery often have little or no experience with clefts, and they are often unable to offer as much aid or advice as parents would like. I've written this book because I believe that parents are motivated and capable of understanding more about their children's clefts.

Parental anxiety is rooted in the unexpectedness of this birth event and a lack of information about the cause and nature of the cleft. Your concern may be compounded by not knowing how to go about feeding your infant or coping with the many subsequent problems associated with the management of clefts. *The Cleft Palate Story*, combined with the assistance of parent support groups and trained professionals, is designed to allay your anxieties by describing how the condition can be managed and a successful outcome facilitated.

The principal aim of this book is to provide information in a clear and positive format to reduce your anxiety over the unknown consequences of cleft lip/palate treatment. With the help of this book, you can reassure your child so that he or she will be better able to handle the many examinations, medical procedures, and hospital admissions required. With more information, you and your family will understand that the treatment plan developed by the cleft palate team means that things are moving toward a successful conclusion: your child's cleft and its physical and psychological effects are going to be well-managed.

This book is a practical guide—it starts from the moment you are told that your child has a cleft to the rehabilitation options available. It is designed to help you cope with the impact of your child's facial disfigurement, which can in most cases be readily made only temporary. The book begins with a typical hospital scene at the time of the birth of a child with a cleft and moves on to explain the best feeding methods, the different cleft types, and the causes of clefting. It describes clinical management, including surgery, orthodontics, and speech and hearing rehabilitative techniques. One of the most useful features of the book is an extensive appendix of resources addressing, among other things, when and how to get help with insurance, how to find support groups, and the numerous cleft-related publications and videos available. In sum, *The Cleft Palate Story* is a comprehensive work, generously illustrated to provide you with important information about the many ways to help your child.

In describing the types of cleft lip and cleft palate, their causes, and their long-term management, this book should help you understand clefts and help you make the most-informed decisions for your child. The portrayal of treatment sequences will help you understand the objectives that the expert clinicians wish to achieve. Ideally, you should review the material with a professional from a cleft palate team who has a complete grasp of your child's treatment program. Because of the great number of rehabilitative steps available to treat the various cleft types, it is not feasible to review them all in one volume. However, several of the surgical-orthodontic treatment options are presented in detail. All make eminently clear that even in the most difficult cases successful treatment outcomes can be achieved.

Extensive efforts have been made to ensure that the treatment strategies described conform to the standards set at most cleft palate clinics at the time of this book's publication. However, constant changes in information resulting from continuing research and clinical experience, reasonable differences in opinion among authorities in the field, and unique aspects of individual clinical situations require that you exercise individual judgment when considering any clinical decision.

Because of the nature of the subject, this book unavoidably contains some technical sections and medical terms that may be hard to understand on first reading. Every effort has been made to explain everything in lay language, except where it is not possible without oversimplifying the subject. If, after reading the book, you have further questions or need clarification, seek the help of a professional on a cleft palate team or the help of a member of a parent support group. One purpose of this book is, in fact, to encourage consultation and communication between parents and specialists.

Acknowledgments

I would be remiss not to pen a few lines conferring credit where it is due. I was privileged to have been trained at what was then known as the Cleft Palate Clinic, University of Illinois School of Dentistry, now the Center for Craniofacial Anomalies at the University of Illinois School of Medicine in Chicago. There I acquired a master's degree and wrote a thesis on cleft palate under the supervision of Dr. Samuel Pruzansky, Director of the Cleft Palate Clinic. Our professional relationship continued for another two decades, during which time we coauthored a number of scientific papers. Dr. Allan G. Brodie, Chairman of the Department of Orthodontics at the University of Illinois School of Dentistry, challenged me to remain active in cleft palate research and associate with Dr. D. Ralph Millard, Jr., a plastic surgeon in Miami. Doing so helped answer many of the questions involved in what is perhaps the fundamental issue related to cleft treatment: the influence of growth and surgery on palatal and facial development.

Our surgical team made up of Dr. D. Ralph Millard Jr. (plastic surgeon), Dr. Tony Wolfe (plastic and craniofacial surgeon), and I (orthodontist) succeeded in achieving a high level of facial esthetics, speech normalcy, and dental alignment. Dr. Bernard Fogel, Dean of the University of Miami School of Medicine, Dr. Reuben Rodriguez-Torres, Medical Director of Miami Children's Hospital, Ambassador David Walters, President of the Miami Children's Hospital Foundation, and Allan Applebaum from A. S. Beck Securities and Alpha Omega Foundation all provided emotional and financial support that helped make possible our team's facial and palatal growth studies. To all of them, I owe deep thanks and much gratitude.

I extend thanks to my office staff including Claudia Roberts, Lourdes Figueroa, Leslie Phipps, Gillian Kelley, and Maryland Jacobson for their typing of the manuscript and organizational skills, to Anne Belmonte and Francis Fink for their excellent cast photography, to Dr. Lin Hu, who performed many of the lateral cephalometric tracings, and to Nick Crespo for developing, organizing, and performing many of the three-dimensional cast analyses; were it not for his untiring efforts, the serial cast studies could never have been accomplished. My appreciation to Bruce Henderson for his editorial suggestions.

Also, special thanks to: Little, Brown and Co. for giving permission to use some photographs published in *Plastic Surgery of the Facial Skeleton* by S. A. Wolfe and Samuel Berkowitz (1989); Childbirth Graphics of Rochester, New York, for the use of excerpts from "Expressing Breast Milk"; and New England SERVE Regional Task Force on Health Care Financing for the use of excerpts from "Paying the Bills: Tips for Families on Financing Health Care for Children with Special Needs."

Immeasurable thanks are likewise due to my many colleagues in the American Cleft Palate Craniofacial Association and in various cleft palate clinics worldwide, including Europe and Asia, for having contributed to my understanding of cleft lip and palate management and to them, too many to recognize by name, I shall be forever grateful for their professional knowledge and personal friendship.

My professional growth has been nurtured by my understanding wife, Lynn, who made it possible for me to spend endless uninterrupted evenings at my desk while at the same time encouraging me to "stay with it." And warm hugs to my two daughters, Beth and Debra, for their endless expressions of support and love.

I cannot say enough for those countless children with various palatal and facial clefts whom I have treated over the past three decades, and to their parents—to all of them this book is dedicated. In their enduring perseverance and fortitude, my young patients and their fathers and mothers have taught me much about the human spirit and the joy that can spring from surmounting nature's adversities.

*I*ntroduction

When a baby is born with a cleft, the questions parents ask most frequently are:

- Can the cleft be surgically repaired?
- When can it be repaired?
- What will my child look like when he or she grows up?
- Will my child be normal in other respects?

The short answers to these questions are, in most cases, reassuring. In correcting a cleft, the long-term objectives are to achieve normal jaw growth and thus normal facial form and appearance, normal speech, normal hearing, normal chewing and swallowing, and psychological well-being in that the child should act like any other well-adjusted child.

Be aware, however, that an effective treatment program takes time and requires the use of a variety of procedures. In the broadest sense, the treatment of children with clefts involves more than surgery—a number of specialists are available to treat potential problems in such areas as hearing, speech, orthodontia, and psychosocial adjustment. It is important to emphasize that the timing and type of surgical and orthodontic treatment procedures for cleft lip/palate can vary not only according to the needs of the child, but also in relation to the experience of the clinicians involved. Other procedures can be as effective as those described in this book. Furthermore, to state it plainly, you should know that not all physicians, dentists, orthodontists, nurses, speech/language pathologists, plastic surgeons, and oral surgeons are qualified and experienced in treating cleft lip or cleft palate. If there are any questions to which you cannot get answers, or if you simply need further explanation, seek out a member of a specially trained cleft palate team, or call the American Cleft Palate Craniofacial Association's Cleftline (1-800-24-CLEFT) for a list of cleft palate teams and support groups in your area. Keep in mind that although there are usually solutions to the physical problems involved in clefts, it may take some time to achieve the desired results, because the way the palate and face grow will determine the best time to perform surgery and other corrective procedures.

Three different cleft types are presented to show the excellent changes in appearance that occur after surgery. The final result, however, is usually achieved in the teen years after a number of surgeries to the lip and nose.

Incomplete Unilateral Cleft Lip

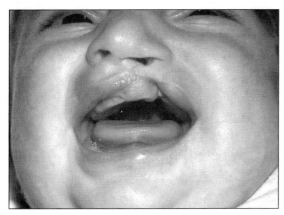

Child at 16 weeks.

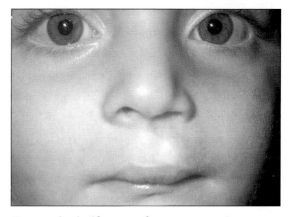

One and a half years after corrective lip surgery, which was performed at 5 months of age.

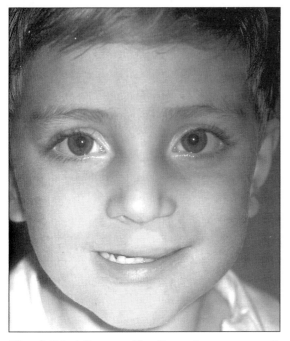

The child at 3 years. The lip and nose are well aligned. Additional lip and nose surgery is usually necessary to improve facial esthetics.

Bilateral Cleft Lip and Palate

Case 1

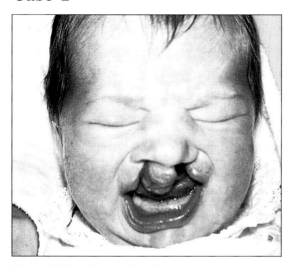

The child at 1 month of age.

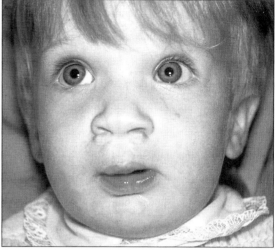

After lip surgery, at 17 months of age. The upper lip is still being pushed forward, but this characteristic will improve with growth.

Case 2

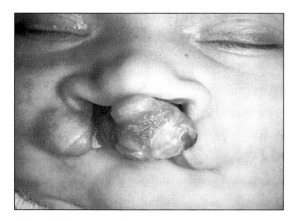

The child at 3 weeks.

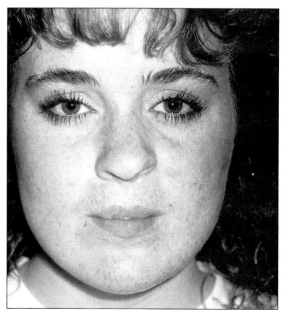

At 12 years. The child's upper lip appeared to be pushed forward for her first 10 years, but with orthodontic treatment and natural facial growth, the facial contour became more normal.

Unilateral Cleft Lip and Palate

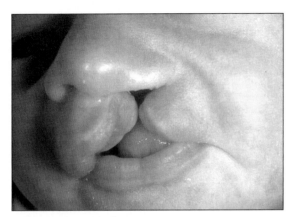

The child at 10 days.

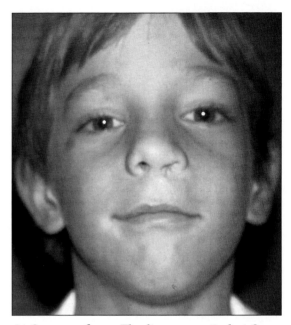

At 6 years of age. The lip was united at 2 weeks and the palatal cleft closed at 18 months. Additional surgery to the left nostril will be performed at a later age.

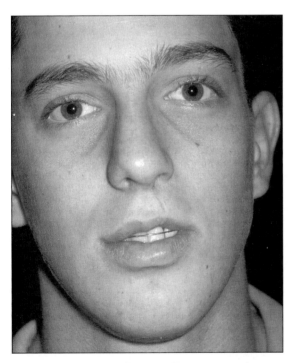

At 16 years. The left nostril was revised at 10 years. Additional lip surgery will be performed to lengthen the left lip segment.

Unilateral Cleft Lip and Palate

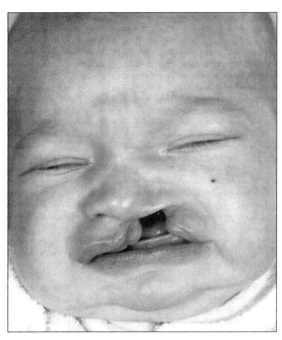

The child at 3 weeks of age.

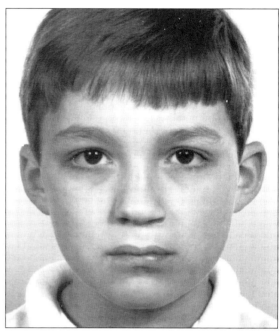

At 5 years of age. The lip was united at 3 weeks of age.

CHAPTER 1

When a Child Is Born with a Cleft

The birth of an infant is an event of profound psychological significance. The relationship of the parents to each other, and their feelings and attitudes to the coming of the child, can influence the significance of the birth. Because the birth of a baby with a cleft is usually unanticipated and because the hospital personnel involved in the delivery have probably little or no experience with clefts, the birth of the affected baby is likely to assume crisis proportions and set a chain of events into motion.

The parents realize something is wrong as soon as they hear the pauses and the modifications in conversation about their baby's status. Unfortunately, there is usually a delay before they are told about the defect and shown the baby. This interval, filled with dreaded anticipation of what the baby will look like, is very difficult to bear. The parents feel hurt, disappointed, even resentful and inadequate. With skilled and thoughtful professionals in the hospital, such feelings can give way to more positive ones as the mother and father are assured that the cleft is not life-threatening, that they will be able to care for and feed their infant, and that the outlook for a happy and normal life for their child is excellent.

Coming Home

Upon leaving the hospital with your newborn, you must of course assume responsibility for its feeding and care. You will benefit by the advice and counsel of an actively involved qualified professional or a parent trained by a parent support group. Be on guard, however, against well-meaning relatives and friends who may betray strongly held opinions and prejudices about clefts and their causes. These are usually based on error, superstitions, or folklore, the latter sometimes including imagined parental misdeeds. Help educate them about cleft palate and encourage them to be involved.

The bonding process between mother, father, and infant begins with psychological attachment to the newborn. This is important for the child's growth and development. Physical contact between mother and infant immediately after birth not only initiates the attachment of mother to infant, but facilitates maternal feelings as well. Become physically familiar with the cleft by touching it, if you haven't already. Becoming familiar with it will help you feel less ill at ease about it.

Parents as Partners

The effect of having a child born with a cleft is in most ways no different for fathers than it is for mothers. This is a reflection of the fact that as our society has evolved, male-female roles have become blurred. Fathers now assume a more active caretaking role in the parenting process, and they have become more sensitive to their children's needs. Robert Guessford has written that when a child is born with a birth defect, most fathers experience a myriad of feelings: grief, depression, weakness, guilt, anger, frustration and isolation, among others.* Every aspect of being a father becomes magnified. To counteract these difficulties, Guessford suggests that fathers be included in every aspect of their child's treatment. Support groups run by involved fathers, or for fathers exclusively, may go a long way toward eliminating the feeling of isolation.

Relatives and Friends

As your child grows and becomes aware of the cleft, the reactions of those around can greatly affect his or her ability to deal with the condition. Such social reactions become particularly significant as the little boy or girl grows into school age, with the accompanying desire to be accepted. Therefore, advise family and friends to treat your child as they would any other child. Don't be over-solicitous or overprotective.

In an era when the public is being increasingly educated about the needs and feelings of the handicapped, such new awareness and sensitivity must surely extend to the children with cleft lip and/or palate. Ridiculed for centuries as "harelips" whose intelligence was questioned, those who happen to have clefts must now be recognized as being normal in every other respect—and accepted as such, be it on the school playground or in the workplace.

Clefts are repairable, and their effects on speech and other functions are treatable over time. However, even those with clefts who have not had the opportunity for treatment should not have to suffer

*From *AboutFace*, vol. 6, no. 4, July/August 1992. For more information about The National Father's Network, contact: James May, Project Director, Merrywood School, 16120 NE Eight St., Bellevue, WA 98008, tel 206 282-1334.

the additional stigma of public ridicule. So if your child comes home one day and tells you that he or she has been called a "harelip" in school, sit down with your child and explain that babies born with a physical difference, such as a facial defect, may represent a chance occurrence, "a quirk of nature." Stress that your child is normal in every other way and if a problem, such as difficulty in speech, is present it can be corrected to some degree. However, in the same way that a child with poor eyesight must continue to wear eyeglasses, the child with a palatal cleft may continue to speak a little differently. Explain to your youngster that although the term "harelip" was used years ago because the united lip resembled a rabbit's lip, today it is not in good taste to use this word. Point out that in most cases the corrected lip can be made to look almost natural, although some scars may remain.

In terms of intelligence, the afflicted child is no different than any other child whose IQ will vary with the general population. Studies have shown that children with clefts perform similarly on IQ tests as their brothers and sisters and that clefts are not a sufficient foundation upon which to draw conclusions about intelligence. Children born with the most severe clefts have become physicians, dentists, nurses, movie actors, engineers, teachers, successful businesspeople, and even speech pathologists. As with any congenital disability, the parents must help the child learn how to cope with some special problems as he or she grows into adulthood. Consultations with experienced psychologists can help parents better understand their own feelings and how best to interact with their child. The child with a cleft should be treated as any other child, with the knowledge that there may be some problems that require special handling.

When Your Child Asks About the Cleft

As your child grows and begins to ask about the lip scars, provide simple and truthful answers geared to your child's ability to understand. Providing good answers depends in large part on your understanding of clefts and of the various stages involved in treatment. With adequate knowledge, you will be better prepared to help your child handle problems as they arise. Providing straightforward answers to questions also contributes to better communication between you and your child. At the appropriate age, your child can be encouraged to ask questions directly of a designated cleft palate team member who has good communication skills.

Most professionals who understand the meaning of the crisis to parents, who listen to parents, and who offer guidance and support set the stage for building a healing relationship. This leads to a family-centered health-care approach, which enhances involvement for the family members, giving them an opportunity to participate in the decision-making process. Only in this way can parents help their children achieve their maximum health potential.

Your Questions

You may have questions about what caused the cleft, as well as concerns about your child's well-being and future. In trying to find a cause-and-effect relationship, some parents search their family histories for the presence of clefts. Others may review the pregnancy, especially as it relates to smoking, drinking alcohol, or the use of medications. What is known at this time about the causes of clefting is discussed in Chapter 4.

One of this book's principal purposes is to help you cope with having a child with a cleft by providing necessary information and by showing that with a little help your child can live a normal and productive life. Additionally, you are encouraged to ask questions of any member of a professional healthcare staff who is qualified to discuss cleft treatment. This includes parents from parent support groups who have been specially trained. You should expect all your questions to be answered accurately and with sensitivity.

Support Groups

The first months of life of a baby born with a cleft can be the most difficult time for parents. During your child's infancy, you will want information about how others care for their babies with clefts. In addition to the counseling of a cleft palate team and talking with other parents who have a child with a cleft, many parents have joined together at a community level to exchange information and provide mutual emotional support. Most parents find it helpful simply to know how others cope with the problems of raising a child with a cleft.

Support groups enable parents to:

- Talk with adult patients and parents who have a child with a cleft lip and/or palate
- Get practical help from others who share common problems
- Share information about treatment and community resources
- Provide special support for parents of newborns with cleft lip and/or palate

- Educate the public about cleft lip and cleft palate
- Accomplish more than any individual could do alone, such as lobbying for funds from government officials, or undertaking specific fund-raising projects

AboutFace* is an international information and support organization for people with facial differences and their families (toll-free number: 1-800-225-FACE; see also Appendix C). Their chapters and support groups provide face-to-face support. Trained volunteers are available for new parents immediately after the birth of an affected child or after the diagnosis of an acquired disfigurement. Support is ongoing as long as the family wishes it. The group publishes a manual on how to form a parents' support group.

AboutFace, which has offices in Toronto, Canada, and Warrington, Pennsylvania, works closely with the National Cleft Palate Association (for parents and other interested parties) and the American Cleft Palate-Craniofacial Association (for professionals involved in treating people with clefts).

Most support groups are interested in contacting other parents of newborns with clefts who are not yet part of a group. The initial contact person should be trained by an appropriate professional or an experienced parent who is a member of a parent's support group. At group sessions, professionals are invited to present information dealing not only with cleft treatment, but also with the best methods of rearing the child with a cleft and protecting the relationship of the parents to each other. Equally important is the development of programs for teenagers with clefts that include siblings and friends.

*For more information write to: AboutFace, 99 Crown's Lane, Toronto, Ontario, Canada M5R 3P4; 416-944-3223; FAX: 416-944-2488; U.S. Office, 1002 Liberty Lane, Warrington, PA 18976; 1-800-225-FACE; FAX: 215-491-0603.

AboutFace resources include parent support training, books, videos, and a lending library.

Adopting a Child with a Cleft*

Joan M. McCartney, who adopted a Korean infant with a complete unilateral cleft of the lip and palate, wrote extensively on the subject of adopting a child with a cleft. Her pamphlet, "Promising Smiles," deals with many factors involved in nurturing a child with a cleft. The following excerpts compose only a small amount of the useful information contained in this booklet.

As Ms. McCartney writes, the excitement of adopting a child with a cleft is "mixed with questions and concerns beyond those which accompany non-special-needs adoptions." Her pamphlet, which is designed to provide insight on the initial adoption period of a child born with a cleft lip and palate, seeks to lessen the fears that birth defects elicit.

Not for all prospective parents

The presence of a facial/palatal cleft might be a simple challenge to one family and an overwhelming commitment to another. Families who adopt children with clefts or other medical or emotional needs are not special or different. It might simply be that their attitude toward the child's particular handicap is more relaxed. The sum total of unpleasantness amounts to just days when compared with the years of joy that the child brings.

*From "Promising Smiles—Adopting a Child with a Cleft Lip and Palate," written and published by Joan M. McCartney, 21 S. Auten Ave., Somerville, NJ 08876.

Mixed feelings are normal

Both positive and negative emotions are common to all adoptions. Those awaiting the arrival of a child needing medical care naturally have additional concerns. Mixed emotions do not always disappear. Moments of doubt about having said yes to the adoption, or worry about one's ability to meet the challenges of the child's special needs, mingle with feelings of intense excitement and overwhelming joy.

Despite these feelings, most parents agree that they have made the right decision and feel stronger in their ability to parent their wonderful child.

Preparing siblings

Children tend to focus more on the arrival of a brother or sister and all the excitement it entails than on the unique appearance of the baby. Explanations presented in logical and simple terms are usually all that are needed. Just explain that before the baby was born the lip and top part of the mouth did not grow together as they should have; it does not hurt and the doctors will fix it after the child comes home.

Remember—your excitement and joy for this baby will be contagious to your other children. Couple this with the genuine openness that children possess, and your newest child will be welcomed with enthusiasm and loving acceptance by its new big sisters and brothers. Both baby and older children need to be loved and accepted just the way they are, not in spite of the way they look.

Health insurance

It is important to examine your health insurance program to make sure that adopted children are covered in the same way that biologically related children are covered. Pre-existing conditions clauses may exclude the baby's birth defect. If you are switching to a new policy, find out if there is a waiting or grace period. It is important to look into the various state-funded programs available for special-needs children. Most states have Children Medical Services programs whose workers can inform you about available state aid programs.

Handling the Future

Take photographs of your baby. Like any child, your child will want to see proof of his or her beginnings with the family, and a lack of presurgery photos may smack of nonacceptance of the child's differences. Show your baby to family and friends with pride, and don't be afraid to go out in public with him or her before the cleft has been repaired, unless it is an older child who has become very sensitive to stares received in the past. Under these circumstances, take the child on short, quiet outings in less-public areas, or on visits to loving relatives and friends. This will help build the older child's self-confidence.

CHAPTER 2

*F*eeding Your Child

For you and your baby, mealtime is an especially important occasion. Here you make contact and get to know each other; it should be a relaxed and enjoyable experience. Cuddling helps establish a sense of security in your infant. Although your baby has mechanical difficulty in suckling (more with a cleft palate than cleft lip) and will spend more time and effort than the average child in getting an adequate amount of milk, the action of suckling is important for infants for many reasons. This chapter presents the technique recommended by most pediatricians involved in cleft treatment programs for feeding a child with cleft lip and/or palate.

Some of the material in this chapter is adapted, with permission, from "Expressing Breast Milk," by Sarah Coulter Danner, RN, and "Breast-feeding a Newborn with a Cleft Lip and/or Palate," by Joan McCartney, both of which appeared in *Wide Smiles*, vol. 1, issue 3, and in Ms. McCartney's monograph *Promising Smiles*. Additional material was adapted, with permission, from "Get Your Baby into a Routine," by Anne Cassidy, from *Working Mother* magazine, July 1992.

The Feeding Routine

Newborns

Newborns eat and sleep whenever they feel like it. At some point during the first year of life, however, babies and their parents need a routine. This does not mean that your infant eats, naps, and goes to bed at precisely the same time every day, but these activities should take place in the same order and at about the same time each day.

Maybe clocks and calendars are not your thing; maybe you and your infant thrive on disorder. However, if you notice your baby is especially cranky at day's end, you may have to introduce some regularity, even if you could do without it. Alternatively, maybe you're accustomed to a sense of order and control. Then, suddenly, the whims of an infant must be attended to. Don't stop planning your days, but remind yourself, "This is only a tentative schedule. I may not get through everything I had planned." Learning to tolerate more unpredictability will help you and your baby make the necessary adjustments towards establishing a routine.

Finally, there are special cases to consider. Premature babies, for instance, may need regular feedings, and approximately 10% of healthy, full-term babies have immature nervous systems at birth and need the inherent regulation that a schedule provides.

Amount and Frequency of Feeding

After birth, if the baby is being bottle fed, twenty to thirty minutes of actual sucking, with about forty minutes of total feeding time, should be adequate.

Initially, the baby should be fed every three or four hours, or six to eight times per twenty-four-hour day. If he or she falls asleep before finishing a sufficient amount of food, more frequent feeding sessions will be necessary.

As your baby's and your skills improve, the feedings should become shorter, to about thirty minutes per feeding, four to five times per day.

An infant of approximately three months of age should consume about three to four ounces of milk at each feeding. For an older baby, five to six ounces per feeding should suffice (it is always a good idea to have one- to two-ounce portions available for use in emergencies by a babysitter). As thinned solids are introduced at four to six months of age, spoon-feeding is appropriate. Following these standards, normal weight gain (one to two pounds per month) can be achieved in most infants.

Feeding Technique

All infants, with or without clefts, whether bottle-fed or breast-fed, must cover the base of the nipple, or the areola of the breast, with their lips and compress the milk reservoirs. The tongue presses the nipple against the roof of the mouth, forcing the crosscuts in the rubber nipple (the best type of nipple to use) to open, or to draw milk from the mother's breast.

Children with a cleft palate cannot create sufficient negative pressure to suck milk, which is expressed from the nipple between the upper and lower gum pads, because of the absence of a palatal seal. Further, unless precautions are taken, the likelihood of emission of milk or other foods from the nose of these infants is greater. Children with a cleft lip usually only have problems grasping the nipple.

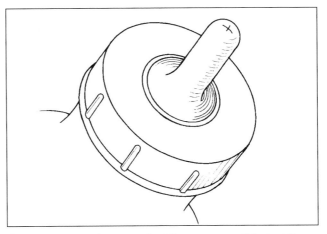

Cross-cut nipples, used with compressible bottles, offer the advantage of controlling the flow of liquid when feeding. Also, because the container must be compressed, you have more control of how much milk your baby is getting. The infant aids the feeding process by gumming the nipple after the lip and the bottle make contact.

Feeding and swallowing patterns in the newborn with a cleft palate are invariably altered. Even small clefts of the soft palate can affect feeding and swallowing. With clefts, swallowing occurs without the assistance of compressive forces produced by pressures built up in the mouth. You may wish to position the infant or child at a thirty-five to forty-five-degree angle to take advantage of gravity to stimulate the swallowing (pharyngeal) reflex. Be aware that feeding techniques for a child with palatal cleft require some modifications from the norm; patience is required. For instance, the infant may swallow more air than usual, and milk may escape through the palatal cleft into the nose.

The baby feeding from the breast and bottle must be burped frequently to expel swallowed air, which can cause bellyaches. If you're breast feeding, alternate between breasts every four to five minutes, burping the infant each time before it resumes feeding.

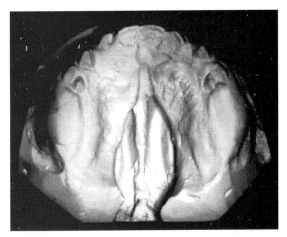

This is a plaster cast of a palatal cleft (roof of the mouth). The cleft space here is large.

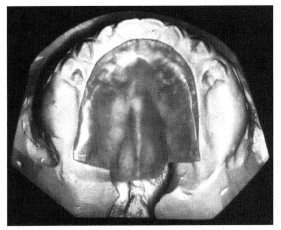

An obturator is a plastic plate that is, in rare instances, used to close off the cleft space. It may have to be refitted as the palate changes shape and size with growth. After each feeding, the plate must be removed and cleaned thoroughly.

Obturators

Some practitioners recommend that a plastic plate (obturator) be worn to block off the cleft space while the child feeds. This plate requires frequent modifications to fit properly as the palate grows. Moreover, it has been found that even in cases of wide palatal clefts, the infant can feed quite satisfactorily without an obturator when the parents are properly instructed in good feeding techniques.

Bottle Feeding

For all new parents, the decision to bottle-feed or breast-feed their newborn is a personal choice. As a parent of a child with a cleft, be prepared for not only the common concerns over adequate physical and emotional nourishment, but also for the additional time and patience needed. While breast feeding is not impossible for the baby with a cleft lip and/or palate, it does require a greater amount of the mother's time and energy because she herself will have to do most of the work of expressing and maintaining an adequate production of milk. Breast milk is, however, best for babies. Bottle feeding, on the other hand, allows both parents to share both the burden and the pleasures of frequent feeding.

How to bottle-feed

To begin feeding, cradle the baby at a thirty-five to forty-five-degree angle to the floor. Direct the nipple toward the inside of the cheek on the noncleft side—not down the throat. Slight intermittent pressure on the bottle, coupled with the infant's gumming of the nipple, will allow for slow and steady feeding. A cross-cut nipple or Playtex nipple, combined with the force of gravity and a compressible bottle, will

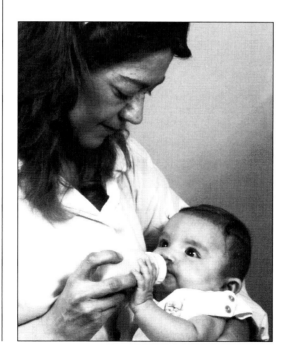

The parent holds the baby at a thirty-five to forty-five-degree angle to the floor, the ideal position for bottle feeding.

usually permit an adequate flow and allow the baby to control the amount of fluid and air being swallowed. If the milk flows easily onto the tongue, swallowing automatically occurs. Feed slowly with small amounts—two to three ounces—at a time. If choking occurs, stop feeding and place the infant's head down slightly below the rest of the body and suction the nose and mouth using a nasal aspirator (Dunlop, Marietta, GA) or a Medibear ear aspirator (Bruder Healthcare, Marietta, GA). Wipe any milk from the face and start feeding again slowly. If the milk still seems to be flowing too fast, the nipple should be replaced with one that has a smaller opening.

Nipples, bottles, and formulas

When bottle feeding a baby with a cleft, the type of nipple and the size of its hole are particularly important. Nipples come in various shapes and sizes. The so-called lamb's nipple is long, the NUK Sauger style is flat, and some nipples have flaps that supposedly act to close off the cleft space. However, lamb nipples

Near right, nasal aspirator used to clear food from the nasal passages should food enter the nose. Far right, an ear aspirator can also be used.

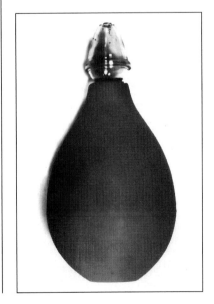
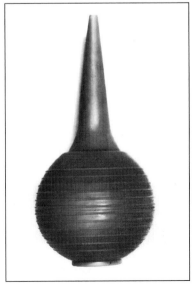

and flap nipples, as well as gavage (tube) feeding and dropper feedings, should be a thing of the past. Gavage feeding should be used only occasionally and for short periods of time, such as after lip surgery to prevent sucking and stress to the lip sutures. A standard nipple with a cross-cut used with a plastic compressible bottle is the most efficient and widely available feeding system. The Playtex nursing system with the pinhole in the nipple and a compressible and disposable plastic bag is an acceptable system because the parent can control the rate of feeding.

Nipples available for the reusable system are: Gerber, NUK cleft palate, and NUK (newborn and regular). Nipples available for the disposable system are: Gerber standard style bulb, Gerber Natural Flex, and NUK.*

The Mead Johnson nurser, the Infa-feeder, and the Playtex baby nurser kit are compressible nursing systems. The Mead Johnson nurser uses a cross-cut nipple and a compressible container. The Playtex Nurser comes in four- and eight-ounce sizes and allows the parent to control the feeding speed. Its plastic disposable bag collapses as the baby drinks, thereby reducing the amount of swallowed air and the subsequent need for burping. A new bottle nipple may be boiled, if necessary, to soften it. The nipple opening should not be so large that the milk runs out rapidly when the bottle is upside down.

Special nursers include the Mead-Johnson cleft lip and palate nursers and Gerber's NUK nursing system with a cross-cut nipple.

---

*NUK and Gerber blind nipples are available only through Gerber Baby Care. They are $1.00 each, including postage and handling. Add your state sales tax to the order, and state the type and style of nipple needed. Send a check or money order to: Gerber Baby Care, P.O. Box 120, Reedsburg, WI 53959-0120. Or charge to your MasterCard or Visa ($5.00 minimum order) by calling 1-800-4-GERBER.

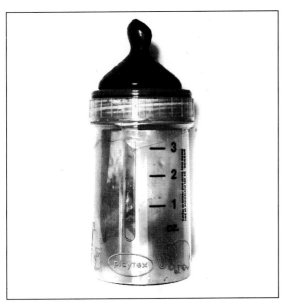

A NUK nipple on a Playtex nurser. This nipple comes with a cross-cut fissure or a pinhole (Gerber, Fremont, MI).

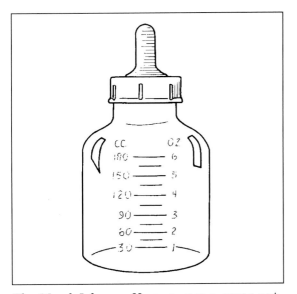

The Mead Johnson Nurser uses a cross-cut nipple and a disposable and compressible container. It can be reused until the container begins to lose its shape, but it must be exceptionally well cleaned.

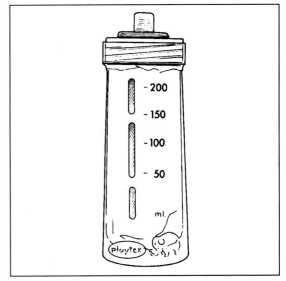

Playtex Nurser. This nurser is useful because it enables the parent to control the feeding speed. The plastic disposable bag collapses as the baby feeds, thereby reducing the amount of swallowed air and the subsequent need for burping. This nipple is adequate because it opens only when the fluid container is squeezed.

While these nursers are designed as disposable units, they may be cleaned and reused. The life of the unit is usually six to twelve feedings. Keep in mind that latex rubber reacts with the baby's saliva and can break down. Direct sunlight can also weaken latex. Latex nipples should be replaced every two to three months or more frequently if the nipple becomes sticky, enlarged, or cracked. The bottle must be discarded if, when you squeeze it, it no longer returns to its original shape. The nipples can be sterilized like other nipples, but do not boil the bottle to sterilize it.

Most of the basic infant formulas in general use (eg, Similac, Enfamil, soybean substitutes) are acceptable for infants with a cleft palate. Discuss the options with your pediatrician.

Modifying nipples

Because of varied formulas in use today, the consistency of your formula may be thick, or, if breast milk is used, thin. If you are not getting the flow of milk you desire, use the following procedure to make the nipple hole larger or to make a hole in a blind nipple:

1. Use a needle that is approximately the same size as the hole size you desire.

2. Heat the tip of the needle in a flame until it's red hot. Make sure the needle is in the flame for at least one minute so that the natural carbon formed on the needle during heating will be burned off. If it is not burned off, the needle will leave a black mark on the nipple that is hard to remove.

3. Immediately insert the needle into the nipple after removing it from the flame. If you're using a NUK nipple, the hole should be made on the side "NUK" is imprinted. Push the needle from the inside out.

4. Push the needle in and out a few times to make sure the hole is complete.

5. Repeat the procedure with a larger needle if the hole is not big enough.

Breast Feeding

There are differences of opinion about breast feeding for infants with a cleft. It is not disputed, however, that breast milk is the best food for infants. Those first trying to breast-feed an infant with a cleft lip or cleft palate may think any difficulties are due to the cleft. Mothers can, in most cases, however, successfully breast feed their newborn, even if the child has a cleft lip. Because the breast itself tends to conform to the shape of the lips, these infants will probably have no more difficulty than other babies in breast feeding

Infants with a palatal cleft, on the other hand, have anatomic problems that may interfere with their ability to suckle adequately. If the infant has no other problems, it is possible to breast-feed. However, patience and modifications in feeding technique will be necessary to provide sufficient nourishment and minimize maternal stress. If you want to breast-feed your infant, get acquainted with the various procedures that can make breast feeding comfortable for yourself as well as for the baby.

How to breast-feed

Breast feeding requires a period of trial and error. To begin, massage the breast before nursing, which allows the milk to flow more easily. Gently massage the base and middle of the breast in one area, stim-

This is one of the ways an infant can be held for breast feeding. It is important that both you and your baby are comfortable. Other positions that work well are shown in *Bestfeeding: Getting Breastfeeding Right for You* (Mary Renfrew, Chloe Fisher, and Suzanne Arms; Berkeley: Celestial Arts, 1990).

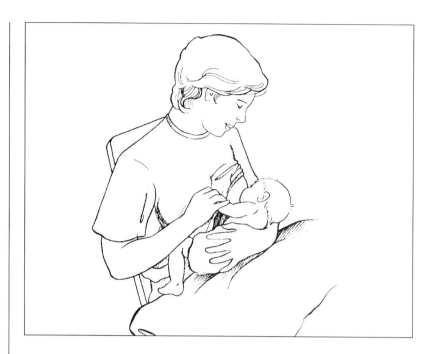

ulating the flow of more milk toward the nipple. Make small, circular motions starting near the chest. Squeeze the breast gently as you slide your hands forward from the chest toward the nipple. When you're ready to feed the baby, compress the areola (the dark area around the nipple) with your fingers so that the nipple protrudes, making it easier for your baby to grasp.

Massage can also be used after feeding to stimulate the breasts to produce more milk. While manual or electric pumps are useful, hand expression of breast milk is just as effective once the techniques are mastered. Massaging and stroking the breast before each feeding helps keep the milk moving to the milk reservoirs. You may also need to increase your fluid intake if you are not producing an adequate amount of milk.

Because breast feeding is not as efficient as bottle feeding, more feeding time is necessary for breast feeding. Each feeding should take up to forty-five minutes of actual sucking time, starting with twelve minutes at each breast. Feed the baby every two to three hours during the day and every four to five hours at night. The breasts are usually replenished in two hours. Frequent nursing (every two to three hours) during the first two weeks of life is often recommended to establish a good milk supply.

If after several attempts the infant cannot hold onto the nipple or he or she does not seem to be emptying the breast, collect the remaining milk and finish each feeding with the collected milk in a bottle. Whenever you supplement feedings with collected breast milk in a bottle, you should still begin each feeding by putting the infant to your breast. This will minimize nipple confusion and keep the baby motivated to continue breast feeding. With increased strength, adaptation, and endurance, breast feeding might become possible over time.

Finally, be patient and realize that longer feeding sessions may be necessary for a baby with a cleft. The infant may tire and not nurse long enough to obtain enough milk to be satisfied.

Breast feeding after surgery

After your child has had surgery, feeding patterns and techniques may have to be changed for awhile. Discuss this with the child's surgeon. If breast feeding isn't feasible, a breast pump to extract the milk will be necessary. It is essential to use a squeezable bottle and a proper nipple to control the milk flow. After a few days, occasionally offer your breast to your child, but don't expect immediate success. Acceptance will occur with time. Be patient. Placing a little breast milk on the breast nipple before feeding will help remind your infant what needs to be done.

Breast feeding after hard-palate surgery may be discontinued for a short while. Surgeons usually have different preferences, so it's a good idea to talk to your surgeon. The baby may even refuse the breast for a week or two. The breasts must be pumped during this short period to relieve any discomfort and to maintain a proper milk supply. The baby can drink this expressed milk using a bottle or cup.

Electric pumping

Some mothers with infants with clefts choose to express their breast milk. Those with uncomfortably engorged breasts may gain some relief by pumping their breasts. Mothers of premature infants are encouraged to provide their own milk because it contains colostrum and is especially suited to the needs of their babies. A breast pump also helps in situations when breast feeding is temporarily interrupted, such as when the infant suffers from jaundice or when either the mother or child is hospitalized. Also, working mothers may need to use a pump to collect milk while they are away from their infants, and so may women who are under great stress and in whom there may be a reduction in milk flow.

When you first use the pump, start pumping at the lowest pressure level and increase the pressure toward the normal setting until the milk streams out. Start with three to five minutes alternately at each breast. Alternating frequently allows the release of milk in one breast while stimulating the release of milk in the other. Massage the resting breast to keep the reservoir filling. Work your way up to five to eight minutes on the pump for each breast, for a total of twenty-five to thirty minutes. Relax and drink a lot of juice or water to stimulate milk production. Stop pumping if the nipples become sore.

It is recommended that pumping be performed every two to three hours while awake, and only once during the night for a total of fifteen to twenty minutes on each breast as long as a reasonable stream of milk is elicited.

Storing breast milk

Breast milk can be refrigerated for no longer than seventy-two hours, but breast milk left over after feeding your child can be re-refrigerated for up to nine hours. Refrigerate expressed milk in a sterile container; plastic bottles or Pyrex glass containers are most convenient.

Breast milk can be stored for up to two weeks in a freezer compartment within a refrigerator, up to four months in a separate freezer compartment, and six months to two years in a deep freezer. Freeze milk in one- to four-ounce amounts that can be thawed quickly to reduce waste. Frozen breast milk should never be heated in boiling water or in a microwave oven because important elements found in healthy milk will be destroyed. Thaw the frozen breast milk under lukewarm, running water while shaking the container.

Support

When trying to breast-feed an infant with a cleft, get as much support as possible. You may also want to talk to another mother who has gone through this experience. Feeding pamphlets are available from:

La Leche League International
9616 Minneapolis Avenue
P.O. Box 1209
Franklin Park, IL 60131-8209
1-800-LA-LECHE

Childbirth Graphics, Ltd.
2975 Bri-Hen Townline Rd.
Rochester, NY 14263
716-272-0300

Cleft Palate Foundation
1218 Grandview Ave.
Pittsburgh, PA 15211
412-481-1376

As Your Child Grows

Three months to six months of age

At this stage, your baby may eat six times a day, but at least the meals are often at the same six times. He or she may not be sleeping through the night yet but is getting there. Many infants sleep from five to nine hours by this point, much to their parents' relief. Settled infants usually have a drowsy period in the morning and in the afternoon. Waking up, eating, and going to bed at regular hours is important because it helps children synchronize their circadian rhythms—daily fluctuations in body temperature, hormone release, and other functions.

By six months of age, your child can understand that a soothing night-time routine—which includes a story, lullaby, or other calm activity—means that the day is done. Putting your baby to bed while it's still awake helps it learn to fall asleep on its own. If your baby cries, check him or her at regular intervals (every five to fifteen minutes the first night; every ten to twenty the second night), so the child doesn't feel abandoned and so you know he or she's okay. Don't be surprised if this is one of the hardest things you've ever done. It is—but it works!

Six months of age

At this stage, breast milk or infant formula alone is inadequate. Now your baby begins eating solid foods, if he or she hasn't already, enjoying three or four regular meals a day and becoming more and more a full-fledged member of the family. It's necessary to add infant cereals and strained fruits and vegetables to the baby's diet. The baby can now hold up its head to accept or reject food and can swallow and digest semisolid foods. As the child begins to scoot, crawl, or walk, it will get tired and may welcome naps and bedtime more readily than before. Remember, don't give the child a bottle with milk, juice, or any sweetened liquid while he or she is lying in bed. With the baby sucking on the bottle in a prone position, the sweetened liquid will coat the teeth, causing cavities.

In the second six months of life, the "average" baby will probably have several growth spurts, erupt anywhere from two to eight teeth, and catch a cold or two. Any of these can disturb the sleeping and eating patterns you've so carefully nurtured.

Cleaning the cleft

The cleft is not a wound, and it is not tender to the touch. However, if food is left to accumulate in the cleft area, it will mix with mucous secretions from the mouth and nose to form a hard crust. If such a condition has formed, use a soft cloth or gauze that has been soaked in warm, clean water to remove the crust. This problem can often be prevented or alleviated by giving the child a half cup or full cup of water after each feeding, which will eliminate or reduce the buildup of uneaten food. Call the doctor if there is persistent crusting. If dryness becomes a problem in the cleft lip, it should be kept moist by applying baby oil, mineral oil, or Vaseline.

Food-Related Allergies

Allergic rhinitis is the most common allergic disorder in childhood in the U.S., affecting between 10% and 20% of all children. It can cause swollen nasal membranes and chronic nasal obstruction, leading to a change in the way the face grows. Since some children with clefts may have a reduction in nasal air flow (because of a deviated nasal septum and a narrowed nasal chamber), it is important to prevent any further increase in nasal blockage brought on by food allergies.

Symptoms of allergic rhinitis commonly occur between the ages of five and ten years with the peak between ten and twenty years, but there have been reports of allergic rhinitis in infants as young as six months. Symptoms tend to decrease after the age of thirty-five.

Allergy to bovine (cow's) milk is probably the most common food allergy seen in children, particularly during infancy. Sensitivity to bovine milk can lead to vomiting, diarrhea, abdominal pain, and skin rashes; it can also cause nasal stuffiness, coughing, laryngeal swelling, and bronchial asthma.

Food allergy may be one of several causes of irritability in infants, and milk allergy has been documented to cause excessive waking and crying in some. (It is not clear whether such irritability is due to colic or to a direct effect on the central nervous system.) Because the symptoms associated with food allergy can be caused by other types of childhood problems, food allergy is frequently misdiagnosed.

The basic treatment for food allergy consists of eliminating suspect foods from the diet, in consultation with a physician. Milk-sensitive infants are provided with an appropriate substitute formula, which can be their sole diet up to six months of age.

Soybean formula is the most commonly used milk substitute. Alternatives include enzymatically hydrolyzed bovine case formula, such as Nutramigen by Mead Johnson.

CHAPTER 3

The Anatomy of Clefts

Knowing something of the anatomy of clefts is an important first step in understanding and communicating with the specialists on your child's treatment team. Understanding all the variations that can exist in cleft anatomy will make the treatment picture come together better and will make you less uncomfortable about the surgical and orthodontic treatment procedures that your child will undergo. While the anatomy of clefting is not really complicated, the terms will probably be unfamiliar to you. Take some time to learn the terms and concepts presented in this chapter, and refer to the glossary at the end of the book (page 201) when you need to.

The Normal Palate

The roof of the mouth is also the floor of the nose. It is made up of a bony (hard) section, which is composed of two parts. The *primary palate*, or *premaxilla*, is the front part carrying the four upper front teeth (also called the central and lateral incisors).

A View of the Palate, or the Roof of the Mouth

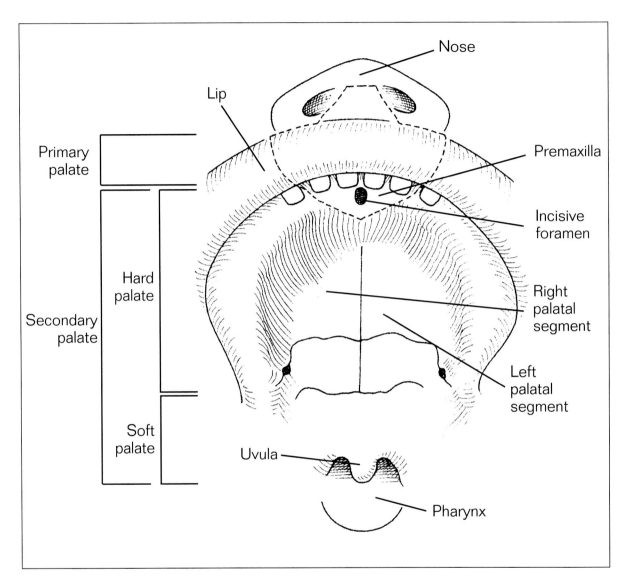

The dashes outline the portion of the lip and the palate that develops separately from the hard and soft palate. *Unilateral clefts* of the lip occur on one side or the other along the dotted line through the lip and possibly the palate. *Bilateral clefts* of the lip occur on both sides of the incisive foramen and include the lip segment called the *prolabium* (the part of the lip attached to the premaxilla). (Adapted from Millard, Ralph D., Jr. *Cleft Craft*. Boston: Little, Brown, 1977.)

The *secondary palate* is the bony area behind the primary palate containing the rest of the upper teeth. These bones on the right and left are also called *lateral palatal segments*. These bones normally fuse together in the middle during the first nine weeks of fetal development.

The soft palate (as distinguished from the hard or bony palate) and uvula are muscles attached to the rear of the hard palate, and during speech they act together as a valve separating the mouth (oral chamber) from the nose (nasal chamber). The uvula, which can be seen dangling at the back of the throat, is a small muscle at the back end of the soft palate. Together, the soft palate and uvula control air flow and prevent food from entering the back of the nose.

The Face and Palate with a Cleft

Clefts of the lip and palate involve primarily muscular and bony parts of the face, mouth, and throat. A cleft of the lip and/or palate occurs when the lip elements and the right and left palatal segments fail to come together within the first nine weeks of a fetus's development.

It is important to distinguish between complete and incomplete clefts of the lip and palate because the extent and location of the lip and palatal cleft determine the degree of facial distortion seen at birth. *Incomplete* clefts of the lip have intact skin and muscle between the lip and the nose. This band means less distortion brought on by abnormal muscle pull. In *complete* clefts of the lip, the cleft extends through the entire length of lip to the floor of the nose. The abnormal muscle pull distorts the nose extensively and creates wide clefts between the lip

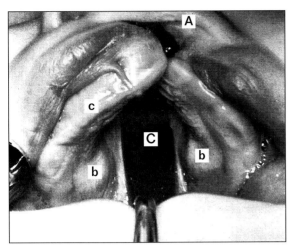

Close-up view of a complete unilateral cleft lip and palate. The outward pull of the cleft musculature causes distortion of the nostril (A) and lip. Note right and left palatal segments (b) and alveolar ridge (c). (C) indicates the cleft palate.

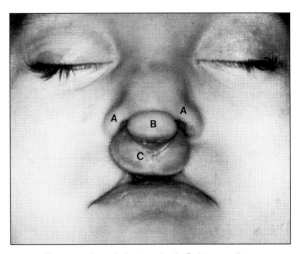

An infant with a bilateral cleft lip and a protruding premaxilla (C). (B) indicates the prolabium.

segments. In complete clefts of the lip and palate, the lip and palatal segments are pulled in abnormal directions by the separated muscles, causing the lip and nose to appear to be broader and flatter than they would be in incomplete clefts.

When complete clefts of the lip involve the hard and soft palate as well, wide separation of the right and left lateral palatal segments occurs because of an absence of an attachment of the palatal segments with the vomer (the partition that separates the nasal chamber into two parts). The protruding premaxilla in complete unilateral and bilateral (one- and two-sided) clefts of the lip and palate is carried forward in the facial profile by an overgrowth of the bone attaching the premaxilla to the nasal septum. The premaxilla in incomplete bilateral clefts of the lip does not extend as far forward in the facial profile as it does in complete bilateral clefts. All of these problems can be corrected with surgery, time, and subsequent growth, which is essential to the corrective process.

Variations in clefts

As children differ because of their variable and individual endowments, so may their clefts show differences. Normal growth adds yet another dimension to the malformation, because it alters the cleft and its associated parts, either simplifying or complicating treatment.

There is great anatomic variation in the types of clefts. The anatomic classification system for clefts is based on the location, completeness, and extent of the cleft. Since the lip, alveolus (tooth-bearing area), and the hard palate develop from different embryonic sources, any combination of clefting can exist. Clefts of the hard and soft palate alone (isolated cleft palate) may vary in shape and length, extending in various degrees to the area just behind and between the two central incisors.

At birth, the cleft palate, nostril, and the nasal chamber are distorted by the outward pull of the muscles of the lips and cheek around the cleft. Should the hard palate be cleft, the tongue will enter the cleft and push the palatal segments apart as well. As a result, the width of the nasal chamber on the cleft side will increase.

The noncleft palatal segments may be attached to the vomer (the part that separates the nasal chamber into right and left halves) and, therefore, be in a relatively normal position. Alternatively, the cleft segment is detached from the vomer and is pulled outward by abnormal muscle pull of the surrounding cheek and lip muscles.

Uniting the lip musculature in complete clefts of the lip and palate will reduce nostril and palatal distortion by causing the lip, nose, and palatal segments to move together into a more normal relationship.

The degree of initial palatal displacement seen at birth is not related to the ability to bring the palatal segments into ideal alignment; that is, the widest clefts at birth with highly separated palatal segments can still be brought into good alignment by surgically uniting the cleft lip, and by using extraoral (outside the mouth) elastic forces or an intraoral (inside the mouth) plastic plate.

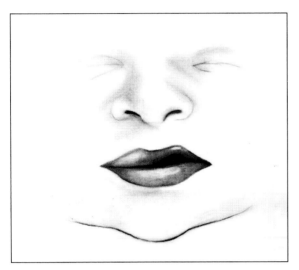

Incomplete unilateral cleft lip.

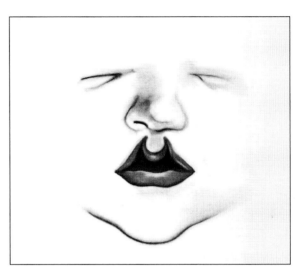

Incomplete bilateral cleft lip.

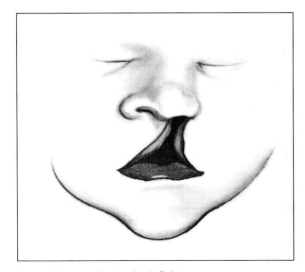

Complete unilateral cleft lip.

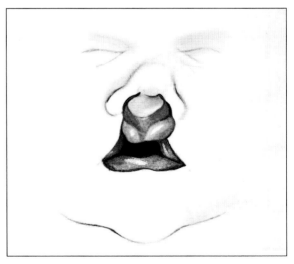

Complete bilateral cleft lip.

Primary Palatal Clefts

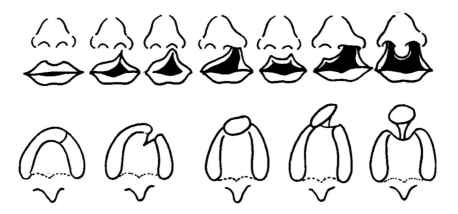

Secondary Palatal Clefts

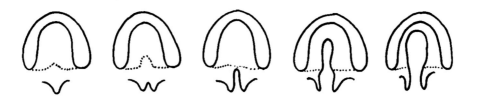

Shown are the variations in the main types of clefts. Top row, primary palatal clefts. Far left, normal lip. The clefts may involve the lip only or may include the alveolus (tooth-bearing area) as well. The cleft can extend toward the nostril on one or both sides. Middle row, the cleft of the alveolus can extend to the incisal papilla on one or both sides to any degree (roof-of-the-mouth views with top as the *front* of the mouth and bottom as the *back* of the mouth). Bottom row, secondary palatal clefts. From left to right, no cleft of the uvula; cleft of the uvula with a submucous cleft of the hard palate (outlined with dots); cleft of the soft palate and uvula; isolated cleft palate (two shown). The cleft involves the soft and hard palate up to the incisal papilla to various degrees.

Combined Palatal Clefts

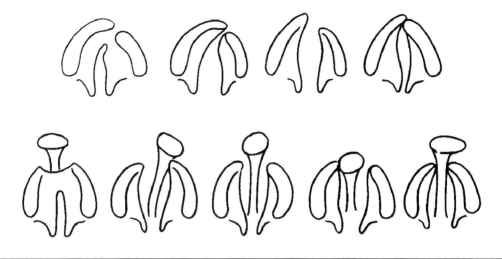

Combined palatal clefts, roof-of-the-mouth views with top as the *front* of the mouth and bottom as *back* of the mouth. In both unilateral (one-sided) and bilateral (two-sided) clefts of the lip and palate, various palatal relationships can exist depending on the completeness of the cleft. Note that when a complete bilateral cleft alveolus exists, the premaxilla projects forward. Ultimately the premaxilla will be repositioned within the arch by orthodontics.

The Causes of Clefting

Clefts of the lip and palate have been documented as far back as the thirteenth century, and they most certainly existed earlier. Clefts can be caused by a number of factors that affect the mother early in the first trimester of pregnancy. These factors include infections and toxicity; poor diet; hormonal imbalance; and genetic interferences. Some of the causes may be due to excessive amounts of cortisone, insulin, vitamin A, aspirin, and a diet deficient in folic acid. Some believe that in very rare instances pressure against the upper jaw by the embryo's knee or the mandible or tongue may cause clefting.

Facial clefts are among the most common congenital malformations in humans. Most geneticists believe that genetic and environmental factors, that is, those things that the mother might have eaten or not have eaten or may have been subjected to, such as measles or other diseases including high fever, can result in a cleft of the lip and/or palate. However, in any individual case a wide variety of causative agents and metabolic factors can be responsible. Good maternal and prenatal health care is essential to increase the possibility that the child will be free of birth defects.

Approximately 7% of live-born children in the United States are affected by birth defects involving the head and face. With a current rate of 3,250,000 live births per year, this means that 227,500 American babies are born every year with either major or minor birth defects of the head and face. The most common of these defects is the cleft lip and/or palate, which affects approximately 1 in 750 births or 4,300 newborns in the U.S. each year. Recent studies show an increasing incidence, particulary over the last century.

Cleft lip with or without cleft palate and cleft palate without cleft lip rank as the third and fifth most frequent congenital malformations in the United States. An isolated cleft of the palate is seen less frequently and has an incidence of 0.4 per 1,000 live births (1 in 2,500 live births). Clefts of the lip with or without a cleft of the palate affect more males (and occur in 1:1,000 live births), while clefts of the palate only affect more females (and occur in 1:2,500 live births). Left-sided clefts (70% of unilateral clefts) are more common than bilateral clefts of the lip and palate, and the right-sided clefts are the least common.

The incidence of clefts of the lip and/or palate varies by racial and ethnic group. The highest incidence occurs among Native Americans (approximately 1 in 278 live births). Among whites of European extraction, approximately 1 in 750 live births will have a cleft lip or palate. Among African-Americans, it is much lower, occurring in approximately 1 in every 3,330 births.

No single factor can be found to be the cause of all facial-palatal clefts. Most can be classified either as an isolated birth defect presumed to be *multifactorial* (meaning with multiple genetic and environmental factors combined) or as part of a genetic *syndrome* (meaning two or more birth defects with a specific natural history and expected course of progression).

Genetic syndromes involving clefts of the lip and/or palate can be considered part of a single gene disorder (autosomal-recessive, autosomal-dominant, or sex-linked), the result of a *teratogenic agent* (anything that interferes with development, such as chemical substances that enter the mother's blood stream and then the fetus's) or event (for example, one induced by hemorrhage, medication, or drug), or one aspect of a chromosomal disorder.

Genetic and environmental factors affect the development and function of humans starting from the time of fertilization and continuing through the prenatal and postnatal periods and throughout life. The critical period during which genetic and environmental events can adversely affect lip and palate development is the sixth through ninth weeks of pregnancy.

For quite some time, most cases of cleft lip and/or palate have been considered to be examples of multifactorial inheritance. Only 3% of cases were previously thought to be of a different cause (syndromic, single gene, or chromosomal). Recently, a number of investigators have found that a significant number of their patients with clefts have syndromic conditions (meaning more than one malformation) that are associated with other anomalies. Specifically, 44% to 64% of the patients with oral-facial clefting are found to in fact have associated anomalies. In 1970, when only 3% of cases were felt to be syndromic, only about fifty clefting syndromes were well described. Today, clefting is known to occur in more than 250 syndromes, including Pierre Robin syndrome, Stickler syndrome, de Lange's syndrome, Marfan syndrome, Gorlin syndrome, and some craniosynostosis syndromes.

Much has also been learned about the ill effects of teratogenic agents. A number of agents previously thought to be of high risk (such as antihistamines that were once used to combat nausea and vomiting during pregnancy) have not been substantiated when subjected to scientific scrutiny, while a number of agents have been clearly identified as being associated with clefting (eg, the fetal hydantoin, fetal alcohol, and fetal trimethadione syndromes). It is imperative that women in their reproductive years be aware of and heed the advice of health-care professionals with access to teratogen information systems. Women must become aware of any medications or drugs they are using or chemicals to which they may be exposed. Because the early critical period of potential cleft formation is at a time before many women are aware that they are pregnant, true prevention will finally depend on an atmosphere conducive to more aggressive preconception health care and counseling. The latest advances in *microcytogenetics* (very small-cell genetics) have helped to better identify a number of chromosome anomalies (abnormal development) associated with clefting syndromes.

The chances of having a child with a cleft lip or palate will vary from one family to another depending on a number of factors. For those individuals where the clefting represents an isolated birth defect and has a multifactorial basis, the risk depends on the number of affected individuals in the family: in general, the risk increases with the number of affected relatives (see Table). For other families, the occurrence and recurrence depends on the specific genetic diagnosis and its natural history and mode of inheritance. Because these hereditary factors are variable and complicated, those with clefting in the family should seek evaluation and counseling from a qualified clinical geneticist. Such evaluation can help identify specific potential medical problems associated with one syndrome or another as well as prevent undue anxiety about the risk of recurrence of clefts in future births.

For couples contemplating or expecting parenthood, many choices based on genetic considerations are available. If either has a suspected family history for a genetic condition or has had a child or family member with a birth defect, such as oral-facial clefting, a diagnostic evaluation by a clinical geneticist and genetic counselling are strongly recommended. Prenatal testing using the techniques of chorionic villus sampling, amniocentesis, and ultrasound are able to reveal more and more of these conditions (although not all birth defects can be diagnosed).

For more information and referral sources, contact the National Society of Genetic Counselors, 233 Canterbury Dr., Wallingford, PA 19086. You can also contact your local chapter of the March of Dimes.

The Risk of Giving Birth to a Child with a Cleft*

Studies indicate that about a third of children born with oral-facial clefts have a family history of clefting. In the United States and Western Europe, there is a family history of clefting in approximately 40% of cases, leaving approximately 60% of cases without any known familial occurrence. There is a greater chance of having a child with a cleft if the mother or father, or other siblings (ie, first-degree relatives) have had a cleft. There is less risk of clefting if only the grandparents, aunts, uncles, nieces, or nephews (ie, second-degree relatives) have had a cleft, and even less risk if only first cousins (ie, third-degree relatives) have had a cleft.

Number of affected parents	Number of affected siblings	Cleft lip with or without cleft palate	Isolated cleft palate
–	–	0.12%	0.05%
–	1	4%–5%	2%–3%
1	–	2%	1.7%
1	1	13%–14%	14%–17%
2	–	13%–14%	14%–17%
–	2	13%–14%	14%–17%
2	1	20%–25%	25%–50%
2	2	15%–50%	50%

*From David DJ, Henriksson TG, Cooker RD. *Craniofacial Deformities.* Australian Cranio-Maxillo Facial Foundation, 226 Melbourne St, North Adelaide, South Australia 5006.

CHAPTER 5

*T*he Cleft Palate Team

Depending on its extent, a cleft of the lip and/or palate usually affects other functional areas in your child's development. Problems may arise pertaining to feeding, facial appearance, speech, hearing, dental functioning, and psychosocial development. All of these problems can be managed best by bringing together many specialists in related disciplines to review the physical and psychological changes involving the cleft and to coordinate treatment to the best advantage of the patient and parents. Your newborn's attending obstetrician, pediatrician, nurse, or social worker may—if they are involved with a cleft palate team—be sufficiently well-informed to outline the general problems for you and provide guidance.

The best time for the first team evaluation is within the first few days or weeks of your baby's life. However, referral for team evaluation and treatment is appropriate for patients of any age. Treatment teams will give you information about recommended treatment procedures, options, risk factors, benefits, and costs to help you make decisions on the child's behalf and prepare the child and yourselves for all recommended procedures.

Often the family is referred directly to a plastic

surgeon, who recommends that the child be examined by other cleft palate team specialists. The team then meets periodically for a cross-specialty discussion of your child in order to exchange information and decide on the appropriate treatment plan. As a parent, you should be given the opportunity to ask questions and to discuss the child's proposed treatment with all of the specialists after your child has undergone a number of diagnostic tests. (A special breakdown of diagnostic tests and procedures can be found at the end of this chapter.)

Who Is on the Team?

The ACPCA (American Cleft Palate Craniofacial Association) states that a cleft palate team should consist, at minimum, of a plastic surgeon, a speech pathologist, and an orthodontist. However, the team may also include a prosthodontist, pediatric dentist, oral and maxillofacial surgeon, general dentist, psychiatrist, audiologist, geneticist, neurologist, neurosurgeon, radiologist, psychologist, otorhinolaryngologist (ear, nose, and throat doctor), social worker, public health nurse, and pediatrician. The team leader can be any one of these professionals, and all team members should possess appropriate credentials and experience in the evaluation and treatment of patients with cleft palate and other craniofacial anomalies.

Each specialist has an important function in assisting both you and your child. For example, the psychologist can, through evaluation of family dynamics, assess the psychological effects the cleft is having on your youngster as well as on your family and friends. Subsequently, appropriate help and support can be offered on a short-term basis or on through your child's development.

Care should be coordinated by the team but should be provided at the local level whenever possible; complex diagnostic and surgical procedures, however, should be restricted to major centers that have appropriate facilities and experienced care providers.

A Partnership—Parents and the Cleft Palate Team

A university/hospital cleft palate team can help you understand and manage the problems that your child will have. Such team guidance can help you arrive at realistic expectations about your child's facial growth and development and about what the team can accomplish during each stage of treatment. Through good communication with the team, a bond can be established that will help both you and the team carry out your individual roles, to the benefit of your child.

In many or most cases, parents and cleft palate team members work together for several years as the infant grows into childhood and adolescence. During that time, you as parents will play many roles, including that of unofficial but important members of the team. You will act as a two-way communications conduit, providing a continuing flow of information about your child to the health-care providers, while, at the same time, helping your child understand and accept the medical treatment. You will also make decisions for your child when he or she is too young to do so. At times, you may be asked to agree to various treatment plans, the technical details of which you don't completely understand; or, alternatively, the technical details are clear, but the necessity or advantages of the proposed treatment are not. It is essential to ask questions of your child's health-care providers at times like these, not only to alleviate your own anxiety but also to enable you to offer reassurance and support to your child.

An excellent source-book for parents and team members alike, entitled *Family-Centered Care for Children with Special Health Care Needs**, eloquently spells out the philosophy behind parent-team collaboration:

• This philosophy recognizes that the family is the constant in the child's life while the service systems and personnel within those systems fluctuate.

• The professional must share unbiased and complete information with parents about their child's care on an ongoing basis in an appropriate and supportive manner.

• This new philosophy recognizes family strengths and individuality and respect for different methods of coping. It also encourages parent-to-parent support groups.

The role of the psychologist and social worker

Your child's habilitation process clearly involves more than medical and dental procedures. The involvement of psychologists and social workers is extremely valuable, and the earlier they become involved, the better. Discussing your feelings as a

---

*Provided by the Family Advisory Board of the Developmental Support Project, U.S. Department of Education, Handicapped Children's Early Program, September 1989; Children's Hospital of Pittsburgh.

parent is important because the team's understanding of family dynamics plays a significant role in developing the most appropriate treatment plan for your child. Discussing your feelings will also be useful for you because you will almost certainly come to understand that the full spectrum of your feelings is normal.

In addition to your family, other factors influence your child's life. For example, the psychologist and social worker will consider the resources or facilities available to him or her in school, in the neighborhood, and in the community. In other words, the child's treatment plan will depend in part on the resources and support available.

Once these professionals have spent time with your child, they will communicate with the team of medical specialists what they have learned. In this way, your child will be seen as an individual throughout treatment. In addressing your family's concerns, these professionals truly facilitate the best outlook for your child and for the family as a whole.

Parents Want the Professionals to Know . . .

Listen to my ideas. I have spent many days and nights with my child and am closely attuned to any changes in his condition. I have observations and a perspective worth listening to. Keep me informed when my child is in surgery. Knowing the worst is better than what I might imagine. Give progress reports on how the surgery is proceeding.

Don't give medical advice or opinions unless you are my primary physician or I request it. Your information may be incorrect, incomplete, and disturbing.

Be careful to give accurate information and take the time to answer all of my questions. It takes time to absorb and understand what you have to say.

Do *not* move my child's bed while I am away without telling me before I return to the room. It is very hard to leave my child at any time, for fear of what might happen, and finding my child gone terrifies me.

Tell me as soon as possible if my child's condition significantly changes. Hearing about this ahead of time helps prepare me for seeing my child in his new state.

Give me an explanation if I can't see my child in the Intensive Care Unit or be with him during a procedure. It is easy to imagine all kinds of scary possibilities.

Give me information I need to care for my child at home as early as possible. Instructions in writing, like a booklet with medication schedules, nutrition advice, recommendations from specialists, and so forth, would be very helpful.

Discharge summary sheets are often too brief for the information I need. I need time to review the materials and get my questions answered before going home with my child. Last-minute changes/additions can be made at discharge.

Understand if I am not at the hospital as much as usual as my child nears discharge. This is a time I need to be elsewhere to prepare for my child's return home.

Provided by the Family Advisory Board of the Developmental Support Project, U.S. Department of Education, Handicapped Children's Early Program, September 1989, Children's Hospital of Pittsburgh.

Let me use the equipment I will be using at home with my child while we are still at the hospital. I need to practice with my child where there is backup while I am learning.

Be cautious with your casual comments about my child. You may be sharing new information, and your words carry more weight than you realize. Think about my child as a child first and not as a child with a handicapping condition.

Think about ways my child may be able to participate in research without interfering with his or her normal routines. It is very important that my child experience the activities and rhythms of daily life as other children do.

Don't treat every parent or child you meet as the same. We are different, with different needs, abilities, styles, personalities, and values. Remember that with time we will be able to absorb and understand more.

Don't judge my ability to parent based upon my child's behavior during the stress of a long hospital visit. My child will behave differently here than at home.

See my child as a whole child and not just a diagnosis or an interesting case. Respect my child's dignity.

Assign my child to the floor he/she was on during previous stays. My child will be less frightened, and we will not have to start over with developing relationships with staff or figure out how things work on a new floor.

Look beyond my child's medical needs and remember developmental needs as well. Don't put off attending to my child's overall development. The illness may continue for a long time, and I want my child to develop as normally as possible in spite of it.

Pay attention to the environment my child is in and plan to coordinate the care so as to reduce excessive medical interventions, light, noise, and other unnecessary stressors.

Consider a variety of approaches and resources to help my child. Be open to other people's practices and routines even though they may be new or unfamiliar, and may require a change in the way you do things.

Thank you for treating me as an equal in our partnership for my child's care.

Diagnostic Procedures and Instruments

Following are some of the more common procedures, tests, and instruments used by cleft palate teams to assess the overall condition and development of children with clefts.

Casts. Casts of the palate and the lower jaw are made from impression material that is placed on a tray and in the mouth for thirty seconds. Plaster is put in the impression to make a mold (also called a cast). It is used to study palatal growth and the bite relationship *(occlusion)* between the upper and lower teeth.

Facial and intraoral photographs. These photographs of the face and the inside of the mouth help in evaluating facial form and contour; they also assist in evaluating dental arch relationships.

Cephaloroentgenographs. These lateral and frontal head x-rays, used for studying facial and skull growth, help assess the form of the passage above and below the oral cavity. The views disclosed include the throat (pharyngeal space) and the size of the adenoids relative to the size and shape of the passage above the soft palate leading to the nasal airways (nasal-pharyngeal airway space). They also help determine the form of the cervical spine as well as the size and length of the soft palate. Cephaloroentgenographs provide information about air flow, not muscle movement.

Multiview videofluoroscopy. This procedure yields x-ray images of the upper and lower jaws (from the front, side, and underneath) on videotape. These three views are used to evaluate velopharyngeal function (eg, swallowing and speech).

Nasopharyngoscope. This instrument contains a fiber-optic lens, which is placed in the nose and directed toward the back and top of the throat. It is used to view the larynx, the soft palate, and the movement of the lateral and posterior pharyngeal wall muscles during speech.

Aeromechanical instruments. These are used for measuring air flow during speech, and, from it, the size of the space between the mouth and nose.

Panographic or panorex images. These x-ray images of the upper and lower jaws reveal the presence and form of the crowns of the teeth and their roots, and the relationship of the teeth to each other. They also reveal the size and symmetry of the vertical portion of the lower jaw that hinges to the skull (ramus) and the body of the lower jaw (mandible).

Otoscope. An otoscope is used to visualize the tympanic membrane, which separates the middle ear chamber from the outer ear canal.

Other audiologic (hearing) evaluation instruments. These aid in the detection of hearing disabilities. The detection of such a disability by the physician marks the beginning of a diagnostic process that varies in duration and complexity with the child's age and the nature of the auditory problem.

Articulation tests. A speech/language pathologist systematically evaluates both correct and incorrect formation and production of the sounds of speech. This includes omissions, distortions, and substitutions of normal sounds or compensatory error sounds. Systematic evaluation of the articulation of speech helps ensure complete and consistent analysis of the problems so that effective and efficient treatment can be planned.

Rating scales of speech intelligibility and acceptability. Rating scales are often used by speech/language pathologists and other members of the cleft palate team to score the overall severity of the communication impairment in several categories. Ratings of intelligibility describe how well an individual's speech can be understood by others, whereas ratings of acceptability describe the pleasantness of both the sound and the appearance of speech.

CHAPTER 6

Preparing for Surgery

It is not possible, of course, to do all necessary surgery during the first years of your child's life. Nevertheless, even though time is a friend that will help your child, don't hesitate to proceed with surgery when the right time arrives. Treatment, which is somewhat akin to assembling a jigsaw puzzle, involves putting the various pieces of the cleft problem together in proper sequence, at specific periods of time, drawing on the expertise of appropriate specialists. The orthodontist on your child's cleft palate team can explain the facial changes that can be expected to occur over time. Sometimes, for instance, the bony parts around the cleft need to increase in size through natural growth before the cleft space can be closed surgically. Each patient's special case must be evaluated on its own merits, with the help of periodic diagnostic tests, before the appropriate surgical procedure can be decided.

Obviously, going to the hospital for cleft surgery can be trying not only for your child but also for you and your family. To ease your concerns, contact the hospital and surgeon's office in advance to become acquainted with the hospital's requirements and procedures. Every hospital should have an administrative specialist in its public relations or patients' affairs office who will answer your questions. You will want to know whether parents are allowed to stay overnight in the child's room, the visitation rules for immediate family and others, payment requirements, and where you and your child should go on first arriving at the hospital.

When surgery is decided upon, be sure that the treatment professional handling your child's case spends time with you and your child, going over, candidly, the reasons for the hospital stay and how long the stay will last. Some professionals believe that a child under six years of age should be told of the impending trip to the hospital only one or two days in advance, while older children should be informed one to two weeks in advance. Whatever the timing of the advisory, the reasons for the hospital visit should be clear to your child. If your child asks a question you can't answer, tell him or her that you will try to find the answer. If the hospital permits, arrange for the youngster's favorite toys and bed-clothes to accompany your child.

It is equally important to inform all siblings of the pending absence from home of their brother or sister, and to explain who will take care of them while one or both parents may be absent. Tell them whether they can contact you at the hospital by telephone and, should there be an extended hospital stay, if and when they may visit. Siblings need to feel included.

One cautionary note: an infant with a cleft must be free of upper respiratory infection before surgery.

Some helpful hints to parents preparing their child for surgery have been outlined in an article entitled, "A Parent's Guide to Cleft Palate Surgery,"* by Dana K. Smith, a mother of a child who underwent surgery. What follows is an excerpt.

*From *Parents & Patients Newsletter*, August 1991, vol. XV-3, and published by the Cleft Palate Foundation of Pittsburgh, PA. Pamplet also available from Dana Smith, 1363 Birchcrest Dr, White Bear Lake, MN 55110.

Questions to the Surgeon

1. What are the presurgery requirements (minimum weight, no pacifier or thumb, off bottle, etc.)?

2. Does the child have to be completely off the bottle, or will a tommy tippy cup be sufficient?

3. What problems could cause the surgery to be postponed (teething, cold, ear infection, flu, etc.)?

4. How long will the surgery take?

5. What anesthesia is used?

6. What is used as a painkiller in recovery in the hospital and at home?

7. How long will my child be in the hospital?

8. What is the diet in the hospital and at home?

9. How long will my child have to wear arm restraints?

10. What will my child be feeling immediately following the surgery—how much pain, grogginess, hungriness, etc.?

11. Can the child's tongue or postsurgery teething tear the stitches?

12. Do the stitches dissolve or are they removed?

13. When and how often will the surgeon check postsurgery progress?

14. How long before the child can return to day care?

15. What are the problems and unexpected results that might be encountered at home? What is the likelihood of each? What is a normal postdischarge course of events?

16. What effect will the surgery have on future ear infections?

17. What are the costs for your services? For the hospital? For the anesthesiologist? Total?

Questions to the Hospital

1. Do you have a pre-admission tour and brochure?
2. Will the child have a private room?
3. May parents spend nights at the hospital and if so, what are the sleeping arrangements?
4. Where do parents shower and eat?
5. Can my child wear pajamas from home?
6. Should parents bring child's blanket, favorite toys or dolls?
7. Will the child sleep in a crib or bed?
8. Are there visiting limitations—time, number of visitors?

Questions to Other Parents

1. How old was your child at the time of surgery?
2. How long was your child hospitalized?
3. Did you stay overnight? Describe the accommodations.
4. How did your child adjust to the arm restraints and pureed food?
5. Did the restraints cause problems with sleeping, car seat, falling down and getting up?
6. Describe your child's diet during/after the hospital stay.
7. What was the hardest thing you experienced?
8. Were any of your worries unfounded?
9. Did any unexpected pleasant things occur?
10. Do you have any specific suggestions?

CHAPTER 7

Surgery

In a book of this size, it is impossible to include the many different surgical procedures for the lip and palate that have yielded excellent results. Many dedicated and skillful surgeons have individualized the timing of the surgical procedures according to the patient's age, the size and shape of the cleft, and the individual's facial growth pattern. In some instances, clefts of the hard and soft palate can be closed early (during the first year of life), but sometimes closure of the cleft must be delayed until a later age, after additional palatal growth has occurred.

All clefts of the lip and palate cannot be treated the same way: surgical procedures are not always performed on patients of the same age, and the same surgical procedures can yield different results on different patients. This is due to the differences in the physical condition of the cleft and the child's facial growth pattern (see page 103). The surgeon's clinical experience will determine which of the corrective procedures is best for your child; it will determine the type of surgery, age at which the child undergoes surgery, and whether infant orthopedics (movement of palatal segments using orthodontic appliances) is necessary. This decision is made in consultation with the orthodontist.

The figures on the next page show some of the surgical procedures used to unite the cleft lip. The general principle in lip closure is to bring the separated lip muscle parts into a normal relationship. In closing the hard palate cleft space, the palatal soft tissue covering the bone is moved toward the middle of the palate over the cleft space. The separated muscles that compose the soft palate are joined together either at the same time or before hard palate cleft closure. Additional surgery at a later age will be necessary to improve the appearance of the lip and nose, and in some cases, to improve soft palate function for normal speech.

From birth to adolescence, there are many acceptable surgical procedures for the correction of the lip and palate and the improvement of soft palate function.

The Lip

In cases of both cleft lip and palate, the cleft lip is generally united first, usually during the child's first two to six months of life, depending on the child's health and weight. In some instances, lip surgery may be postponed until after maxillary orthopedics (the movement of palatal segments by the use of appliances) has been performed. If this sequence of treatment is deemed appropriate, the surgeon and orthodontist will explain why. Additional lip revision procedures will be performed as the nasal and surrounding skeletal structures grow and develop.

Before and After Surgery

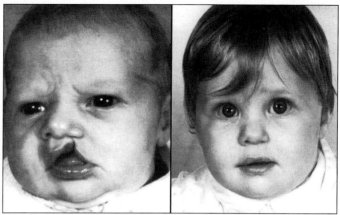

Lip closure for an incomplete cleft of the lip.

At birth.   At 18 months of age.

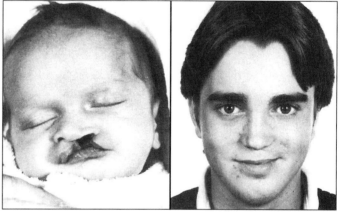

Complete unilateral cleft lip and palate.

At birth.   At 13 years of age.

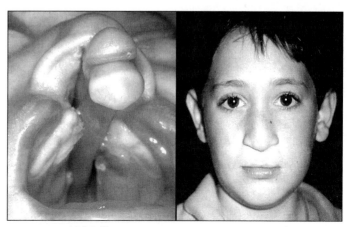

Complete bilateral cleft lip and palate.

At birth.   At 10 years of age.

Logan's bow

This appliance is used to keep the lips together before lip surgery to reduce tension at the suture. The bow is held in place by being taped to the cheeks. The surgical wound is left open for the application of antibiotic ointment and eventual suture removal. The Logan's bow will be kept in place for four to six days after the lip surgery and will be removed with the child under sedation.

Lip adhesion followed by definitive lip repair

Uniting the separated lip musculature reverses the direction of muscle pull, causing the lips, nostrils, and palatal segments to assume a more normal form and contour. The second surgical procedure further improves lip and nose contour. Additional lip and nose surgical revisions are usually necessary at some later age.

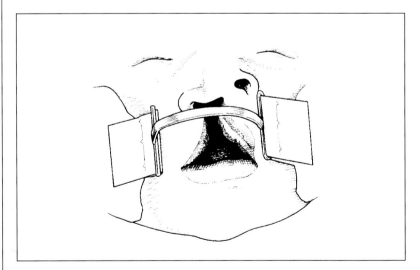

The Logan's bow reduces tension at the suture site in the correction of a cleft. The bow is used to keep the lips together before lip surgery, reducing tension at the suture. The bow is held in place by being taped to the cheeks for 4 to 6 days.

Correcting the protruding premaxilla

Before lip surgery, the protruding premaxilla (the front part of the upper jaw containing the four front teeth) in complete bilateral clefts of the lip and palate can be retruded (pulled back) by using an elastic strap attached to a removable head bonnet placed over the prolabium (the portion of the lip attached to the premaxilla). It exerts a backward and downward force against the premaxilla, reducing its protrusion. This helps the surgeon bring the lips together by reducing the tension at the sutures. The infant wears the elastic band usually for a week or two before lip surgery.

Neonatal maxillary orthopedics

A plastic (resin) appliance can be used in some instances to move the child's palatal segments into a more ideal relationship to each other before lip surgery. This procedure reduces tension at the surgical site and permits the lip to be united in one procedure. The length of time the appliance is worn depends on the treatment philosophy of your child's cleft palate team.

Many surgeons and orthodontists prefer to use either a head bonnet with an elastic band or a lip adhesion procedure to bring the separated segments together before performing definitive lip surgery. Some surgeons or orthodontists may recommend another kind of orthopedic appliance be used to hold the palatal segments in a predetermined position after lip surgery while awaiting additional palatal growth.

Lip Adhesion Followed by Definitive Lip Repair

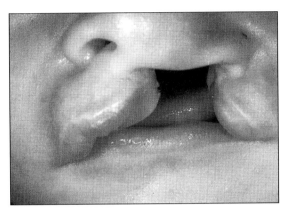

The infant at 2 months of age.

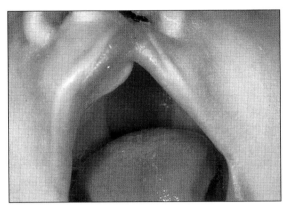

After lip adhesion at 3 months of age.

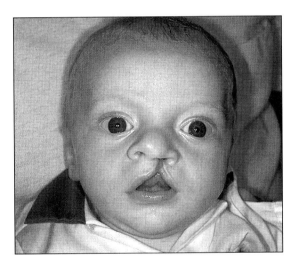

After lip adhesion at 3 months of age, facial view. Lip adhesion is used to unite separated lip elements to establish normal compressive lip forces. This allows the lips, nose, and palate to come together in a normal relationship.

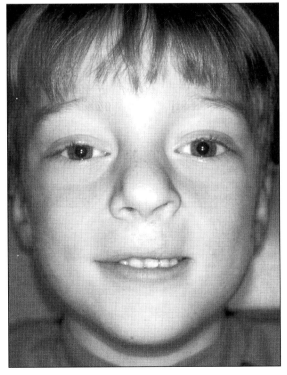

The child at 4 years of age after definitive lip surgery. This surgery aligns the lip elements cosmetically. Future lip and nose revisions will be performed.

Correcting the Protruding Premaxilla Before Surgery

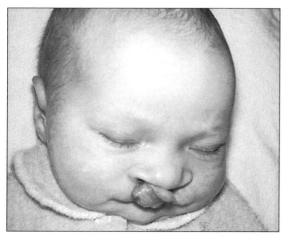

A newborn with a complete bilateral cleft of the lip and palate.

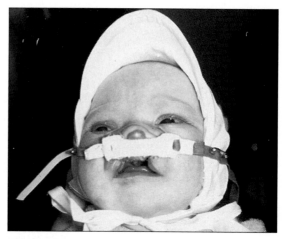

A head bonnet with an elastic strap is placed over the protruding premaxilla. Sometimes the first step used in the correction of the protruding premaxilla before lip surgery, it temporarily bends the premaxilla downward and backward. This is not painful. The head bonnet, which can be worn for 1 to 2 weeks before surgery, is necessary only in cases of extreme premaxillary projection.

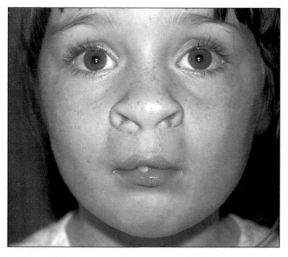

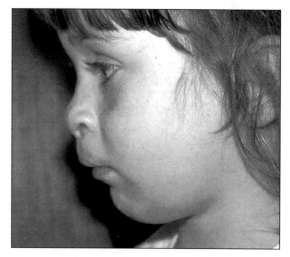

The child 3 years after lip and palate surgery. The upper lip is temporarily protrusive due to the forward position of the underlying premaxilla. The depressed tip of the nose will be surgically brought into normal position at a later age. (See Chapter 8 for a discussion of continued changes in the facial profile with growth.) (Reprinted with permission from Little, Brown and Co.)

Orthopedic Appliances

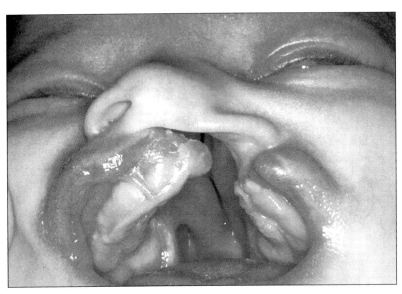

An infant with a complete unilateral cleft of the lip and palate. Neonatal maxillary orthopedic appliances are sometimes used before lip surgery.

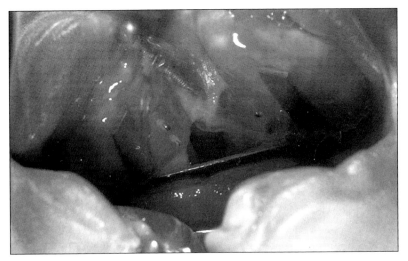

An orthopedic appliance placed on the hard palate to move the palatal segments together before lip surgery. This appliance is one type of many.

The Hard Palate

There are four objectives of cleft palate surgery: to produce anatomic closure; to maximize maxillary growth and development; to produce normal speech; and to establish good dental esthetics and functional occlusion.

The timing of surgery to close the palatal cleft is highly variable. Most clinics seem to favor surgery when the child is between twelve and twenty-four months of age, but sometimes surgery must be postponed until five years of age, or even later, to allow for additional palatal growth.

The surgical procedure used plays an important part in the success of treatment. Balanced are the desirability of obtaining early complete palatal closure and the possible negative effects that extensive surgery may have on the child's palatal and facial growth and development. Although there are many different surgical alternatives, simple closure palatoplasty (palatal cleft closure surgery) designed by von Langenback is illustrated here since it is commonly used today for many types of palatal clefts.

In clefts of the hard palate, the appropriate age for the child to have surgery and the type of surgical procedure used will vary according to the size of the cleft space. In rare instances, the space may remain too large for surgery and require an obturator (a plastic plate) to cover the palatal cleft permanently.

"Push back" palatal surgery

This procedure is an attempt to increase soft palate length while simultaneously closing the palatal cleft space. It may or may not prevent the development of hypernasal speech. Usually a pharyngeal flap (attaching tissue taken from the back of the throat

The von Langenbeck Procedure (Palatoplasty)

Shown are examples of a surgical procedure called the von Langenbeck procedure, or palatoplasty, used to close the cleft space in the hard or soft palate. There are many acceptable procedures to close this space; the von Langenbeck is not necessarily superior to others. These images of different cleft types show how the lining of the hard palate is moved toward the center to cover the cleft space. The age at which a patient undergoes this surgery will vary according to the surgeon's training and experience. Top, complete bilateral cleft lip and palate. The hard palate cleft is closed in two stages. The posterior cleft space (between the lateral palatal segments) is closed first, and then the anterior cleft space, which includes the premaxilla. The cleft of the alveolar ridge (1) is closed later with a secondary alveolar bone graft. Middle, closure of a complete unilateral cleft of the lip and palate. Bottom, closure of an isolated cleft palate. (Courtesy of William K. Lindsay, MD.)

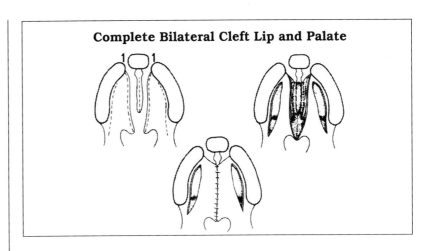

Complete Bilateral Cleft Lip and Palate

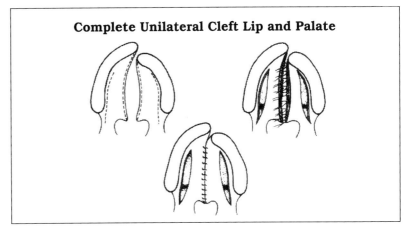

Complete Unilateral Cleft Lip and Palate

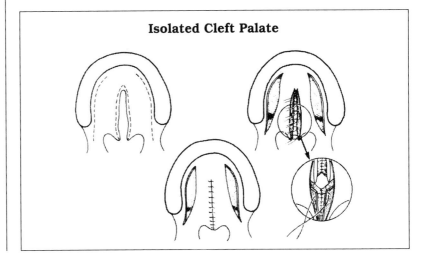

Isolated Cleft Palate

to the soft palate) or a sphincter pharyngoplasty will have to be performed at a later date to control air flow through the pharynx.

The Soft Palate

Surgery to repair a cleft in the soft palate can be performed before or at the same time as surgery on the lip, or it can be postponed and closed with the hard palate. Even after the cleft soft palate muscle is united, additional surgery may be necessary to improve the muscle's ability to adequately close off the nasal-pharyngeal (mouth to nose) opening during speech and swallowing. To be adequate, the functional length of the soft palate must be directly related to the depth of the pharyngeal space (the distance between the posterior limit of the hard palate and the posterior pharyngeal wall). As the soft palate elevates, the surrounding pharyngeal muscles come together by contraction, narrowing the throat's diameter but not completely obstructing air flow.

The soft palate may not be able to make contact with the posterior pharyngeal wall and the lateral pharyngeal muscles for a number of reasons: an exceptionally deep pharynx caused by malformations of the cervical spine (the upper spine related to the neck and attached to the head) that influence its curvature; a short maxilla and/or soft palate; muscle paralysis; and inadequate side wall (lateral pharyngeal) muscle function.

X-ray films of the head will reveal important information about the condition of the above structures, but they will not determine whether the pharyngeal muscles and the soft palate together can control air flow during speech. A nasopharynoscope is the most commonly used instrument to observe the move-

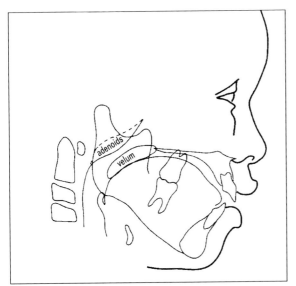
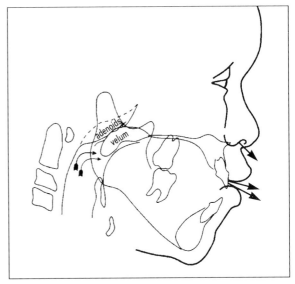

A child's pharyngeal space as seen from head x-ray tracings.
Left and right show good soft palate length and elevation making
contact with adenoids. Right, when vocalizing "you," for example,
the soft palate elevates and makes contact with the adenoids
attached the back wall of the throat. During normal speech, some
air passes on either side of the raised soft palate and enters the
nose. However, most of the air is channeled through the mouth
(arrows) in normal speech.

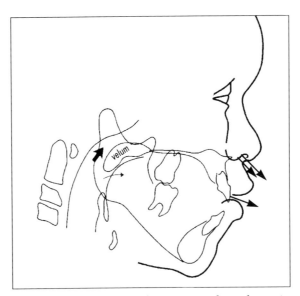

With poor soft palate elevation and inadequate
pharyngeal closure, more air is channeled
through the nose (arrows), resulting in hypernasality.

ments of the pharyngeal (throat) muscles and soft palate during swallowing and speech (see p. 206 for a description of the nasopharyngoscope and how it is used).

The soft palate at rest lies on the back of the tongue. During normal swallowing and speech, the soft palate rises, making contact with the back of the throat. The lateral (side) and posterior (back) pharyngeal muscles, which line the throat, come together and reach the elevated soft palate, closing off the nose from the mouth and creating good velopharyngeal closure. If the soft palate is too short and/or if the surrounding throat muscles do not make contact with the soft palate, an opening that is too large will persist on one or both sides of the soft palate, allowing too much air to escape into the nose. When this condition (velopharyngeal inadequacy) exists, it will result in hypernasality. (Some speech pathologists use velopharyngeal inadequacy, velopharyngeal insufficiency, and velopharyngeal incompetency as synonymous terms). Information derived from nasopharyngoscopy coupled with the results of other diagnostic tests will allow the surgeon to pinpoint how and where the air coming from the lungs is passing the soft palate (velum) and entering the nose. The information will determine where the pharyngeal flap must be positioned to best control excessive air escape. (See pharyngeal flap discussion later in the chapter.)

Changes to the Face and Palate

Since the face with clefting shows results of outwardly pulling and pushing forces, the first goal of treatment is to reverse these forces to bring the skeletal parts into a more normal relationship.

After the lip is surgically united, or after the use of extraoral elastic forces, the outwardly distorted palatal segments are moved together by the compressive muscle forces of the united lip and cheeks. This reduces the width of the palatal cleft by bringing the separated, distorted palatal arches into a more normal relationship. Overlapped palatal segments, should this situation occur, do not create a functional problem or inhibit future palatal growth. The remaining cleft space usually becomes smaller as the bony palate increases in size and moves together.

In clefts of the lip and palate, the distorted nose will appear more normal within the first few months after surgery. However, in children with bilateral clefts, the premaxilla will still protrude until approximately ten to twelve years of age. It must be stressed that midfacial protrusion will be reduced as the face grows and the skeletal parts change in size and their relationship to each other. With additional facial growth, there is an improvement in the premaxilla's relationship to the lateral palatal segments, reducing cleft space size. This in turn will help the surgeon in closing the space at a later age. These palatal and facial changes should be reviewed with the orthodontist (see also Chapter 8). A better understanding of the anatomic changes will reassure you that the facial and palatal distortion seen at birth is only a temporary state that can change and become more normal with time.

After Surgery

After surgery, you will be visited by the surgeon. Your child may be in the recovery room for an hour to an hour and a half until he or she is completely alert. He or she might have a sore throat or sore mouth from the endotracheal (intubation) tube used during surgery. An intravenous (IV) tube may be used for the first day or so of a three- to five-day stay (not counting the day of surgery). Liquid Children's Tylenol may be administered for pain until discharge and thereafter if necessary.

Your child may develop a new pattern of breathing after the palatal cleft is closed, but this usually does not pose a problem. There may be some temporary postsurgical bleeding of the palate, which also should be of no undue concern.

Arm restraints

Different kinds of arm restraints, elbow splints, and immobilizing gowns are available* to prevent the child from touching and damaging the surgical sites. These restraints are used for three weeks, with short periods of freedom so that the child can exercise the arms. A wraparound sleeve with slots into which wooden tongue blades can be inserted is also widely used.

Some doctors stress the importance of wearing arm restraints and adhering to a diet of pureed food. It may be possible to remove the restraints while your child eats, as long as you are there to monitor the feeding. Don't let your child put his or her fingers in the mouth.

As time passes, the arm restraints can be removed for short periods of playtime to exercise arm muscles. Never let the child out of sight during these times. The arm restraints should always be on when your child is sleeping (even napping) or when in the car seat. The arm restraints are usually worn for about four to six weeks.

*Pedi-Wrap by the Medi-Kid Co., PO Box 716, Nuevo, CA 92567, tel 909-928-9528.

Keeping the Child's Hands Out of the Mouth After Surgery

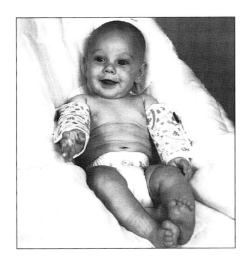 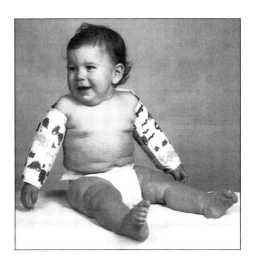

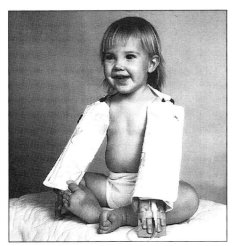 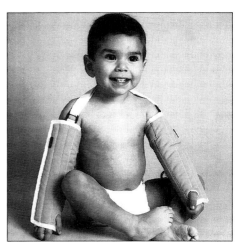

Pediatric arm restraints, which prevent the child from touching the surgical sites immediately after the operation, are worn for 3 weeks with periodic removal for exercise and play.

Feeding after surgery

During the immediate postoperative period, you can feed your infant with a squeezable bottle with a cross-cut nipple to control the flow of formula. For an older baby, cereal or mashed vegetables can be added to the formula feeding. It is hard to prevent the child from sucking on the nipple during feeding, but squeezing the bottle generously enough to satisfy her or him should reduce this sucking tendency. Some surgeons prefer gavage tube feeding (in which the food is pushed outwardly), but then only for a few weeks. A pacifier should *never* be used soon after lip surgery. The external lip sutures are usually removed between the fourth and fifth day.

While your child is still in the hospital, you will be encouraged to visit him or her, especially at mealtimes, to become familiar with the feeding techniques used to prevent the sutures from separating. Each feeding is followed by a drink of water, which serves as a mouthwash. Straws are not allowed for the first couple of months after surgery—this further prevents excessive stress on the lips caused by sucking. The surgeon or nurse involved will discuss all of these procedures, which are designed to help you keep the surgical wound clean and your child comfortable.

Food considerations after surgery are affected by the age of your child and the importance table foods have in the diet. If oatmeal and baby food are still greeted by squeals of delight, you're home free. Otherwise, stock up on a variety of soft foods and foods that can be pureed (a food processor or blender will work fine.) Foods that can be considered are: apple sauce, cottage cheese (pureed), Jell-O, baby food, yogurt without fruit, mashed potatoes and gravy, pureed bananas and strawberries, oatmeal, Malt-O-Meal, Cream of Wheat, Spaghetti-os, soup, milk shakes, pudding, frozen yogurt, sherbet, popsicles, chocolate milk, Slim Fast, juice, and soda pop. You can also puree macaroni and cheese, creamed corn, vegetables, baked beans, and casseroles.

Some surgeons prohibit the use of a spoon to feed the child for the first week. In this case, pureed food in a cup may be preferred. Rinse the child's mouth with water after every meal. It may be several weeks before the bad breath caused by persistent bacteria subsides. There may be a bloody nasal discharge caused by swollen membranes resulting in drainage out of the nose and mouth.

Discharge from the hospital

Most doctors say that once the child is able to manage a full soft diet, he or she can go home. This varies for periods ranging from one to five days after surgery. It may take about ten days for the child to completely readjust to pre-hospital sleep and nap schedules.

Despite adequate planning, be prepared for an unexpected event—a break in the stitches, a pinhole opening in the suture line, or a longer healing process than had been suggested. In about 20% of patients, a follow-up procedure to provide an adequate mechanism for speech may be necessary. The necessity and timing of such procedures will be determined by your child's cleft palate team.

Surgical Treatment After Four Years of Age

Surgery to control air flow to improve speech (by reducing hypernasality) is usually performed around four years of age. Surgical skeletal correction of the midface (upper jaw) and/or mandible (lower jaw) is usually postponed until late adolescence when facial growth is completed. If it is performed while the child is still growing, surgery may have to be repeated.

Additional lip and nose surgery

A number of lip and nose revision procedures may be necessary as the child's skeletal structures and lip muscles mature. Repair of the cleft lip/nasal deformity can be accomplished with limited external incisions on the nose. The timing of nasal surgery may vary.

Pharyngeal flap surgery

If hypernasality is still present after palatal cleft closure, pharyngeal flap surgery is usually the treatment of choice. In this procedure, the lining of the posterior pharyngeal wall is attached to the soft palate, creating a sail-like structure that catches air and food and channels them through the mouth. Depending on its effect on speech, more than one pharyngeal flap revision procedure may be necessary. This surgery may result in a sore throat and neck for a week or so.

Some surgeons prefer a sphincter pharyngoplasty, a procedure that narrows the pharynx. Its proponents claim that it can channel air to the mouth and limit air flow through the nose. With either of these two procedures, extensive speech instruction with parental assistance must follow. Since children learn at various rates and to different degrees, speech improvement may take longer for some than for others and occasionally may even be unsuccessful due to factors not under the speech therapist's or parents'

Pharyngeal flap. If a child has incompetent velopharyngeal closure (too much air escapes into the nose, resulting in hypernasality) by 4 years of age, and the clinicians believe it cannot be corrected by soft palate muscle training, a pharyngeal flap (arrow) is usually the treatment of choice. The lining from the back of the throat is brought forward and joined with the soft palate to create a sail-like flap, which catches both food and air, channeling them through the mouth. Spaces left on both sides of flap (asterisks) permit nasal secretions to enter the mouth.

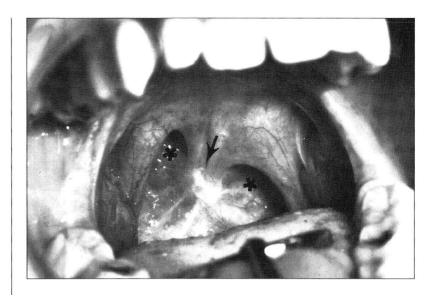

control. Children with clefts can enjoy normal speech, sometimes immediately after palate repair, or sometimes after additional surgical treatments and speech therapy. But for all children with clefts, early stimulation to speak combined with early therapeutic intervention if there are problems will increase the probability that speech will develop normally.

Additional hard palate surgery

The necessity of additional hard palate surgery depends on functional and esthetic considerations: the final relationship of the upper and lower jaws to each other, the presence of alveolar and palatal fistulas (holes), and the size and shape of the palate as it influences the occlusion (the way the teeth meet). All surgical-orthodontic-orthognathic treatment is designed to achieve ideal palatal arch form, normal speech, dental occlusion, facial and dental esthetics.

Adenoids and tonsils

Adenoids (pharyngeal tonsils) are attached to the back of the throat at the level of the hard palate. They vary in size at different ages. They usually increase in size to the time of puberty (typically twelve to fourteen years of age) and then become smaller. The elevated soft palate can make contact with the adenoids during function, helping velopharyngeal closure, the closing off of the nasal from the oral chambers.

If middle ear disease (otitis media) is present, the lateral portions of the large adenoid may have to be surgically removed to unblock the eustachian tube openings to improve drainage of fluids and the equalization of air pressure within the middle ear. The middle portion of the adenoids will be left intact to help velopharyngeal closure.

Sometimes a combination of a shallow pharyngeal depth and a large adenoid will obstruct the nasal-pharyngeal airway, causing frequent periods of waking up at night and snoring. The treatment is a complete adenoidectomy (removing the adenoids). Should the eustachian tubes be blocked, a lateral adenoidectomy adjacent to the openings will suffice. The middle portion is left intact in order not to create velopharyngeal insuffiency.

The palatine (faucial) tonsils are found on either side of the tongue and if they become too large or prone to infection (and if antibiotics are not effective), their removal will be necessary. Very large tonsils may displace the tongue and cause slurred speech, along with distortion in the position of the front teeth. The tongue will be forced against the front teeth, leading to the production of improper speech sounds such as *s* and *th*. In some instances enlarged tonsils may interfere with velopharyngeal function as well, and a tonsillectomy and/or adenoidectomy may be indicated.

A child with a cleft may undergo many surgical and orthodontic treatment procedures. This chapter presents the most common surgical and orthodontic treatment concepts now in use, but it must be stressed that there are many other surgical procedures and orthodontic appliances that can achieve the same results.

The information and images presented here demonstrate that a child born with the most severe facial and palatal clefts can look good and speak and chew well when treatment is coordinated between team members. Treatment involves performing a number of surgical and orthodontic procedures over a long period of time, allowing the necessary facial and palatal growth changes to occur at each stage of development. Although it would be ideal to be able to make all faces look good soon after birth, clinicians today have found that doing too much surgery too soon does not yield satisfactory long-term results. Parents, therefore, need to be patient and cooperative, keeping in mind that time, which is growth, is a friend that can be of great help in achieving excellent results in the child's adolescence and adulthood.

CHAPTER 8

*F*acial and Dental Concerns

Clefts of the lip and palate usually affect a child's dental development. Teeth in the area of the cleft may be missing, and other teeth may be improperly positioned. Because problems with the dentition affect not only your child's appearance, but his or her speech development and chewing ability, attention to your child's dental development is important. Vigilant prevention practices and regular visits to the pediatric dentist will help ensure the best dental outlook for your child. The orthodontist, in conjunction with the rest of the cleft palate team, will devise treatment plans for the best dental and jaw growth.

Primary Teeth

Baby teeth are known as primary teeth or sometimes as deciduous teeth. In a cleft of the lip and alveolus (the bony area that supports the teeth), the primary lateral incisor in the line of the cleft may be twinned (that is, there may be two of the same kind, one on either side of the cleft), or it may be missing, malformed, or normally shaped but not in its normal position. There may also be extra (supernumerary) teeth, as well as malformed and badly displaced normal teeth, all of which may need to be extracted. Most children with such conditions will require orthodontic treatment (teeth-straightening) at various ages, even as early as four years.

The primary teeth usually start coming in (erupting) by six months of age, and by two to three years of age the teeth have fully erupted and are in full function. In some cases, the eruption of teeth may be earlier or later. In either case, dental function will not be affected.

Baby Teeth, Also Called Primary or Deciduous Teeth

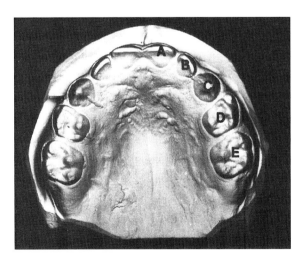 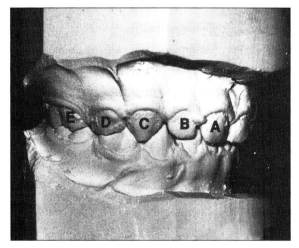

These casts, made from a child without a cleft, show ideal dentition and occlusion (*occlusion* refers to the way the teeth meet). Left, palatal view. Right, ideal occlusion. A, central incisor; B, lateral incisor; C, cuspid; D, first molar; E, second molar. The letters identify the same teeth (on the left and right sides respectively) on both casts.

Permanent Teeth

As is the case with the primary teeth of children with a cleft palate, the permanent teeth in the line of the cleft may be missing, malformed, or displaced from their normal position. While the rate of eruption of baby teeth in children with clefts is similar to that of children in general, the eruption rate of permanent teeth may be delayed. The permanent lateral incisor in the line of the cleft may be missing even though its primary predecessor was present.

Permanent Teeth

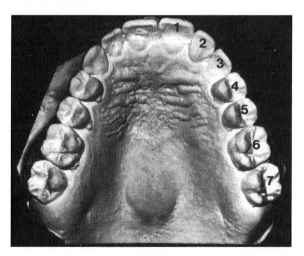 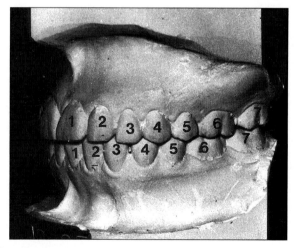

Left, palatal view. Right, ideal occlusion. 1, central incisor; 2, lateral incisor; 3, cuspid; 4, first bicuspid; 5, second bicuspid; 6, first molar; 7, second molar; 8, third molar (not shown). Learning the names of the teeth will help you better communicate with your child's pediatric dentist, general dentist, orthodontist, and oral surgeon. These professionals will, however, use a different numbering system.

Dental Hygiene

Care of the primary and permanent teeth is of particular concern for children with clefts. Such children may have teeth that are poorly formed and therefore they may be more susceptible to tooth decay than other children. Early loss of primary or permanent teeth from tooth decay may complicate therapy and make rehabilitation difficult. Care of primary teeth, therefore, should begin as soon as they erupt.

Removal of dental plaque

Cavities are caused by plaque, a sticky, colorless, bacteria-laden film that forms on teeth and interacts with sugars and starches in foods. As the bacteria break down the sugar and starches, they create acids that dissolve tooth enamel. This is tooth decay. Once the decay penetrates the hard outer surface of a tooth, it can continue to move inward toward the tooth's soft inner pulp. That can eventually lead to the formation of a painful abscess at the root tip, leading to tooth loss.

Don't give a bottle with milk, juice, or any sweetened liquid to your child while he or she is lying in a crib. The sweetened liquid will adhere to the surface of the teeth, causing the beginning of cavity formation. This process is called *crib bottle caries*. Whatever your child's condition, the primary teeth need to be well cared for, by being brushed after every meal. A soft toothbrush with rounded bristle tips is the best type to use to avoid damage to the gums. Replace the toothbrush every three to four months. After your child reaches age two, dental checkups should be made every six months to prevent tooth decay.

Dental flossing

When all the deciduous teeth have erupted, it is important to use dental floss to remove plaque from under the gumline and between the teeth; even tiny brush bristles can't reach those areas. Effective flossing takes practice and patience.

Fluoride

Fluoride works in several ways to inhibit the decay process. Fluoride toothpastes, fluoride rinses, and professionally applied topical fluoride are important sources of fluoride for all children and young adults. In areas where there is no fluoride in the drinking water, your pediatrician or pediatric dentist may suggest a fluoride supplement.

Sealants

One option for helping to protect your child's teeth is sealants. Sealants protect teeth from decay by sealing the biting surfaces of back teeth with a plastic film so the food particles and plaque can't penetrate and break down the enamel. They are designed for children up to the age of fifteen. The dentist usually replaces the sealant every two years although sealants may last for as long as five years.

Seeing the dentist

Schedule regular visits to the dentist for your child from age two onward, even if he or she has no cavities. The dentist cannot do more than the parents in reducing tooth decay and preventing the premature loss of teeth.

Orthopedics and orthodontics

Orthopedics (the movement of bone) and orthodontia (the movement of the teeth) improve chewing, dental and facial appearance, speech, and swallowing for children with clefts. Good dental function also helps protect the bone and gums supporting the teeth from future disease and early loss.

Soon after birth

In some children, the doctor may want to move the palatal segments into a different relationship before lip surgery. This procedure, which falls under the rubric of orthopedic movement, is called *neonatal maxillary orthopedics* (*maxillary* refers to the upper jaw). There are various types of acrylic plates that will accomplish this.

If an infant has a severely protruding *premaxilla* (the part of the upper jaw containing the four front teeth), the orthodontist and the surgeon may wish to retrude, or bring back, the premaxilla by means of an elastic strap attached to a head bonnet before unifying the cleft lip, or by using lip adhesion surgery. Both procedures will reduce lip tension at the surgical site, allow for better cosmetic results after a second lip procedure, and allow for a conservative treatment plan spanning thirteen to fifteen years. Keep in mind that orthodontics will be completed only after the pubertal facial growth spurt, that is, when facial growth is completed. This is approximately thirteen years of age for girls and fourteen years of age for boys. Boys' facial growth may continue into the later teen years, but in most cases, braces can be removed around fourteen years of age. Retainers will have to be worn to replace any missing teeth and to stabilize the corrected palatal arch form.

Orthopedic Correction

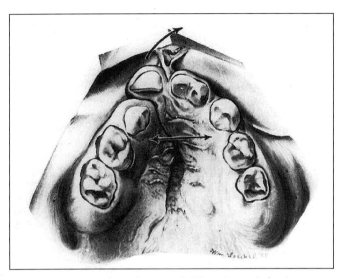

A narrow palatal arch in a child with a cleft places the right (smaller) palatal segment in crossbite. The arrows show the direction that the palatal expander will move the cleft lateral palatal segments.

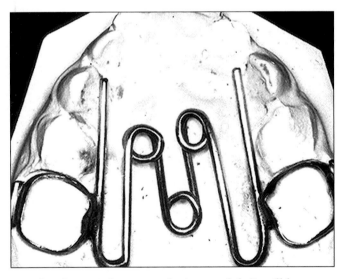

A palatal expander on a plaster model. It will be attached to the teeth and move the segments outward. Children do not find this type of expander uncomfortable, nor does it interfere with speech.

Facial Changes from Birth to Adolescence in a Girl with Bilateral Cleft Lip and Palate

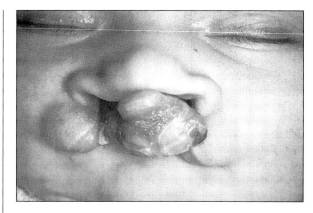

The child soon after birth. The premaxilla projects past the nose, which is distorted. A head bonnet was used to retract the premaxilla and reduce tension at the lip suture before the first surgery.

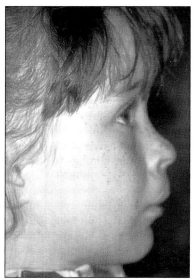

At 6 years of age. The lip was united at 3 months of age. The upper lip is being pushed forward by the protruding premaxilla, creating a convex facial profile. This is a temporary state; the profile becomes straighter as the face grows.

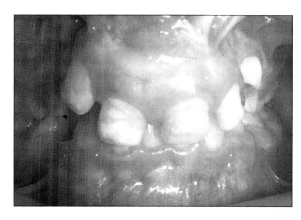

The patient's mouth at 10 years of age. The premaxilla is protruding, creating a severe overjet (the distance between the upper and lower front teeth) and overbite (the distance of the upper to lower front teeth in the vertical dimension).

Shown here are the progressive facial changes as the child underwent surgical and orthodontic treatment. Under the influence of facial growth and orthodontia, the facial profile became flatter and more attractive and the dental occlusion improved. These same facial changes can be expected in most children with bilateral clefts of the lip and palate.

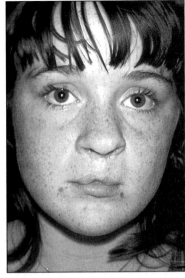 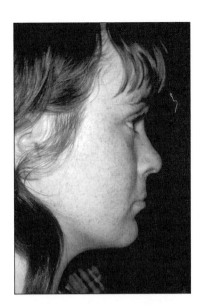

At 12 years of age.

Secondary alveolar bone grafts performed at 8 years of age permitted all four incisors to erupt in proper position. The teeth were then aligned with orthodontia.

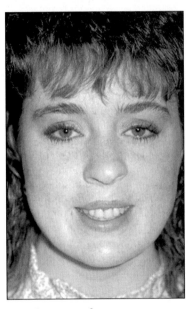 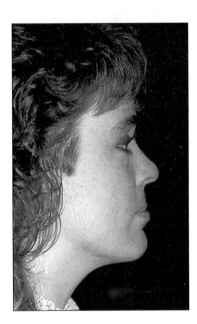

At 18 years of age.

The lateral incisors were made more esthetic with dental restorations. (Reprinted with permission from Little, Brown and Co.)

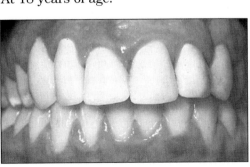

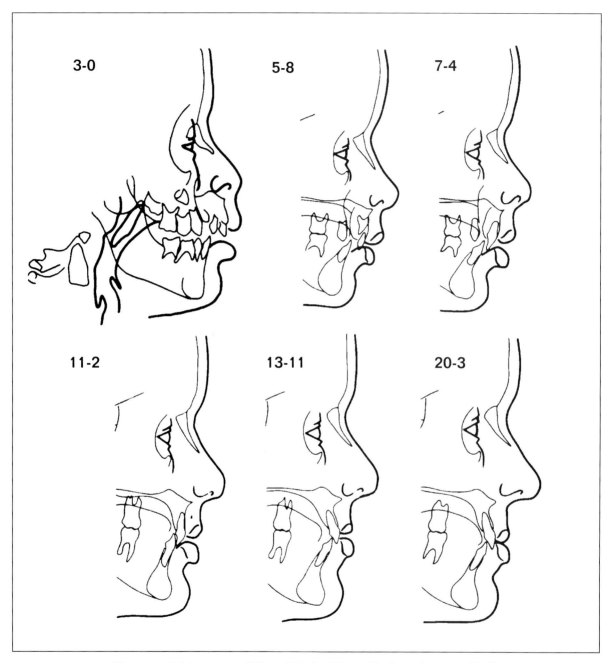

These serial tracings of the girl's facial profile from 3 years (3-0) to 20 years and 3 months (20-3) show a marked improvement in facial esthetics as the face grows. The protruding premaxilla, which carries the upper front teeth and pushes the upper lip forward, becomes less prominent. By 11 years and 2 months, the facial profile is much improved with the front (incisor) teeth in excellent bite relationship. The last tracing (20-3) and last facial and mouth photographs were taken at the same age.

From birth to six years

In this stage, the primary dentition stage, the medial movement of the palatal segments described earlier can place the teeth in each palatal segment into a bad bite relationship (crossbite). The resulting anterior and/or posterior crossbite can be corrected as early as four years of age if the child is able to manage using fixed (attached to the teeth) or removable appliances. This treatment can last for up to one year. This correction is dependent on the movement of the cleft (smaller) palatal segment with its teeth, and not the movement of teeth units per se. To improve dental appearance, a false tooth (to fill the space created by the cleft) is usually attached to a palatal retainer, which maintains the correct arch form. The retainer is worn until the next orthodontic treatment stage.

After the teeth and their palatal segments are properly aligned, *a secondary alveolar bone graft* to the cleft alveolus may be performed by using an autogenous (from the patient's own body) bone graft. While *primary* bone grafting in the past was done at birth, *secondary* alveolar bone grafting is performed any time after the first year of life, usually after six years of age. This procedure is used to replace missing bone in the cleft alveolus (tooth-bearing bone). A cleft of the alveolus usually signifies that bone in that area is deficient, especially if the unerupted lateral incisor is missing.

Secondary bone grafts may be taken from the outer layer of the skull, chin, rib, or hip. They are then placed in the alveolar cleft space. This procedure will: close any remaining fistulas (holes leading from the mouth into the nose); allow the unerupted lateral incisor and/or cuspid to travel through the graft into a more ideal position in the dental arch; and improve the gingival (gum) contour in the area of the missing lateral incisor. There are occasions when

Use of a Removable Retainer with False Teeth and Use of a Bridge

After orthodontic treatment, false teeth may be placed on a palatal retainer. The palatal retainer holds the corrected arch form until a later date when a fixed or removable bridge can be made for the child.

The retainer was worn by this patient for 2 years and then it was replaced with a fixed (nonremovable) bridge at 18 years of age.

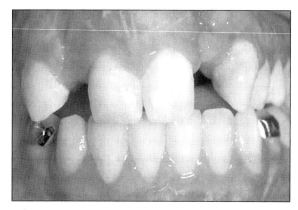

After orthodontic treatment. Both lateral incisors are missing.

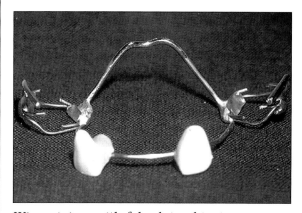

Wire retainer with false lateral incisors.

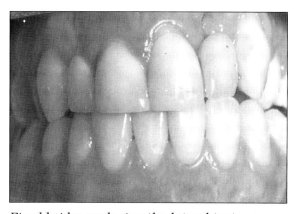

Fixed bridge replacing the lateral incisors.

Secondary Alveolar Bone Graft

The graft is in the tooth-bearing area between the premaxilla and the lateral palatal segments. As the x-ray shows, bone has filled the cleft gap space. A fixed bridge stabilizes the maxillary arch and replaces the missing lateral incisor teeth.

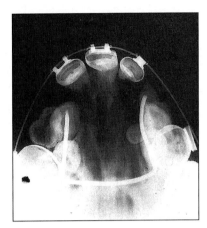

Before surgery.

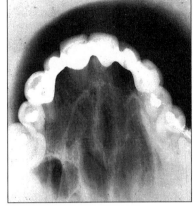

After surgery.

the impacted lateral incisor (which could not have erupted since alveolar bone was missing) will promptly erupt into place after the bone graft. In many instances, however, the lateral incisor may be missing, malformed, or malpositioned. If the tooth cannot erupt, it must be extracted, even after alveolar bone grafting.

From seven to eleven years

In this stage, called the mixed dentition stage, children with clefts of the lip and palate usually have their front (anterior) permanent teeth rotated and out of position. For esthetic and functional reasons, some orthodontists and speech pathologists believe these teeth should be properly aligned before all the permanent teeth have erupted. The corrected anterior arch form also needs to be retained until the final orthodontic treatment stage.

In bilateral clefts of the lip with or without a cleft of the palate, it is easier to correct an anterior crossbite (the upper front teeth positioned behind lower front teeth when the upper and lower teeth meet) while the child is still in the mixed dentition stage and fixed orthodontic appliances can be used. A secondary alveolar bone graft can be performed before or after the anterior teeth are properly aligned with the two lateral palatal segments. Afterwards, a fixed or removable retainer, with or without false teeth, must be worn until the second phase of orthodontic correction in order to keep the teeth from returning to their original crossbite position. The orthodontist, in some cases, will not choose to start orthodontics at this age because the crossbite may not currently interfere with proper chewing and can be corrected when the permanent teeth come in. Crossbites are caused by many factors not under the surgeon's control.

From twelve years on

While this stage can begin earlier, after twelve years is generally the beginning of the permanent dentition stage. Final orthodontic treatment can begin during the mixed or permanent dentition period with a treatment plan very similar to that used for children and adults without clefts. After orthodontic diagnostic records are made (casts of the teeth, x-ray films of the teeth, jaws, and side of the head, and facial and intraoral photographs), a treatment plan will be devised to correct the bad bite (also called *malocclusion*). The orthodontist will describe the treatment plan, the anticipated length of treatment, and the cooperation needed of the child and parents.

Protraction facial masks

A mild midfacial retrusion with an anterior dental crossbite can be successfully treated by moving both the maxilla (upper jaw) and the teeth forward using

Protraction Facial Mask

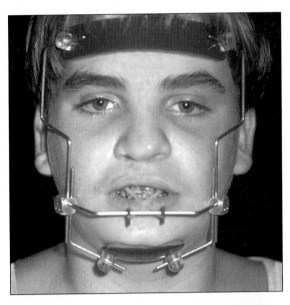

This young man had a unilateral cleft of the lip and palate on the left side, and the upper teeth were in crossbite. A protraction facial mask and elastics (rubber bands) were used to move the upper jaw forward without surgery.

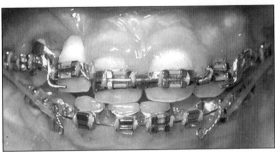

The hooks on the upper arch wire are for elastics, which connect with hooks on the protraction facial mask.

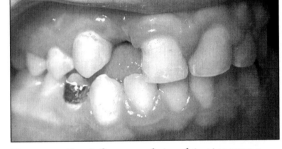

Because the left upper lateral incisor was missing, the cleft space was left open.

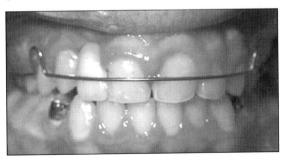

A removable retainer was worn to maintain the corrected arch form. A false tooth attached to the retainer holds the tooth space open and improves dental appearance.

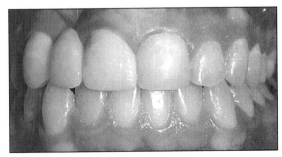

A fixed bridge replaced the removable retainer when the boy was older.

orthopedic (bone-moving) forces. Rubber bands are attached to hooks placed on the upper arch wire at the cuspid and brought to the upper arch wire frame of the mask. In some instances, this treatment can begin in the primary dentition stage, but this depends on the type of crossbite, as well as the cooperation of the child and the parents. It may be advisable to wait until the mixed dentition or the full permanent dentition stage before using protractive forces. The child must wear the appliance twelve hours per day, every day. The best time is 7:00 P.M. to 7:00 A.M. during the week. Although this regimen sounds difficult, most children seem to readily adjust to this schedule. It is not possible to predict the number of months the upper jaw protraction appliance will need to be worn.*

Orthognathic surgery

If your child's upper teeth are in an anterior crossbite due to the retrusiveness of the midface, forward surgical repositioning of the maxillary arch (called, technically, LeFort I advancement by maxillary osteotomy) will be necessary. This procedure places the upper anterior teeth in a proper overbite (vertical) and overjet (horizontal) relationship, and improves facial appearance and dental function.

If the upper jaw is in proper position within the face but the lower jaw is either protrusive or recessive, the preferred surgical treatment will then be mandibular (lower) jaw repositioning to correct the skeletal discrepancy. In some instances, surgery to both the upper and lower jaws may be performed simultaneously.

When a posterior crossbite to one or both palatal segments cannot be corrected orthodontically, surgical widening of the palatal arch will be necessary.

*For further information about the facial protraction mask and its use, contact the Miami Craniofacial Anomalies Corporation, 6601 SW 80th St., Ste. 112, South Miami, FL 33143.

Facial Profiles

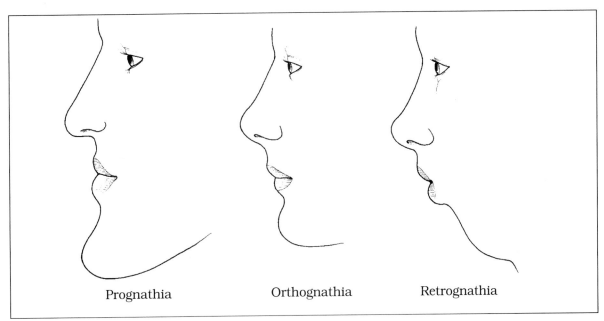

Prognathia   Orthognathia   Retrognathia

Various facial profiles can exist at any age. Retrognathia and prognathia usually require orthognathic surgery. Orthognathia (or mesognathia) can be treated by orthodontia.

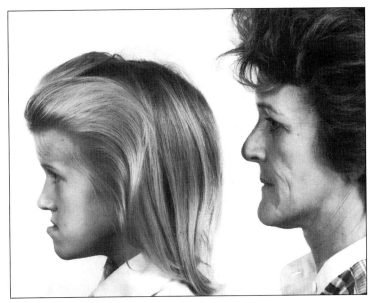

The photograph shows a daughter and mother with a retrusive upper jaw and a prognathic lower jaw.

Presurgical orthodontics, in most cases, will have to be performed before any surgical treatment. After changing the upper-to-lower-jaw relationship, the teeth will have to be orthodontically positioned into a proper bite relationship. This stage of treatment (postsurgical orthodontics) will be followed by the use of a retainer and bridgework (removable or fixed to the teeth) to replace missing teeth and maintain the dental arch form.

Planning orthognathic surgery

It is helpful for parents to have some knowledge of the planning that goes into selecting the proper surgical procedure and how it is carried out in the operating room.

Orthodontic diagnostic records are analyzed to determine the extent of the skeletal defect and to help decide which surgical procedure should be used for its correction. The orthodontist will perform a cephalometric (head x-ray) analysis of the relationship of the upper to lower jaws. The resulting findings determine the direction and the extent to which the upper and/or lower jaws will have to be repositioned. In most cases, some degree of orthodontic tooth movement will need to be completed before surgery is performed.

Just before surgery, a second set of diagnostic records will be taken. Casts that reproduce the upper and lower jaws will be placed in a device called an *articulator* that duplicates your child's current bite relationship. Depending on the extent of the skeletal malformation and what needs to be done to improve it, the upper jaw (palatal) cast will be cut into pieces and the parts reassembled with the teeth of the two jaws in a proper relationship. This trial or "mock" surgery is a rehearsal for the actual surgery to be performed later.

Orthognathic Surgery to Correct Midfacial Retrusiveness

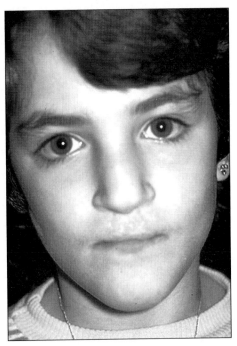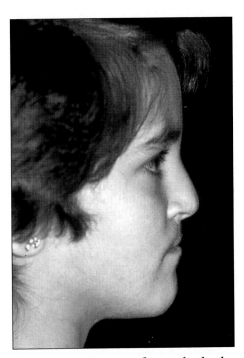

This child had a bilateral cleft of the lip and palate. At 6 years of age, she had a slightly retrusive midface and was developing an anterior crossbite as a result (see below). Wearing a facial protraction mask was not possible for this patient, although it would have been the treatment of choice. Orthodontic treatment was designed to align the teeth in each jaw in preparation for the surgical advancement of the upper jaw. Secondary alveolar bone grafting was performed when the patient was 8 years old.

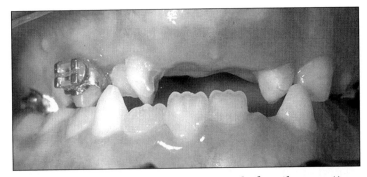

This shows the child's occlusion just before the eruption of the upper front teeth (age 6 years). They erupted into an anterior crossbite, which means they were positioned behind the lower front teeth.

Midfacial Retrusiveness, cont.

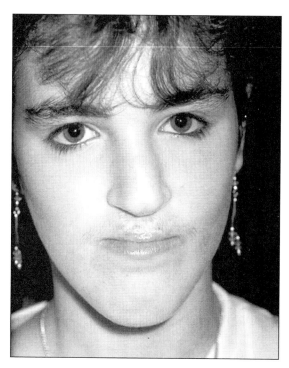 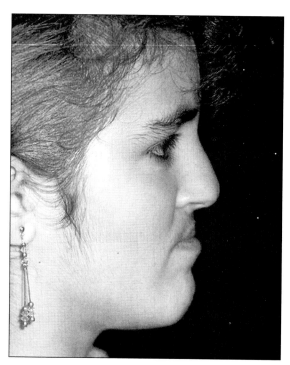

At 14 years of age, she showed increased facial skeletal disharmony between the two jaws. Since orthodontia affects the position of teeth but cannot change skeletal jaw relationships, surgery was the treatment of choice (midfacial protraction treatment was rejected).

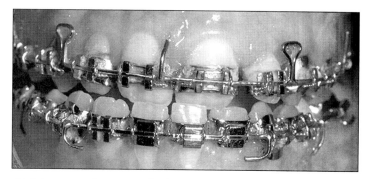

At 14 years of age just before surgery. The anterior cross-bite is still clear.

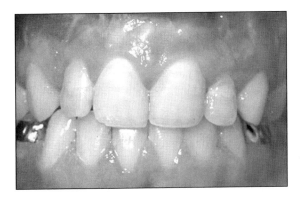

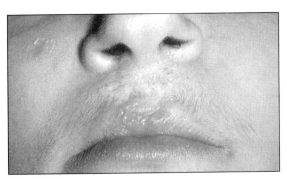

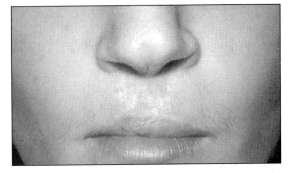

The girl underwent a LeFort I advancement, which moves the entire upper jaw forward. Surgery was followed by 6 months of orthodontia to place the teeth into ideal occlusion.

Before and after lip revision.

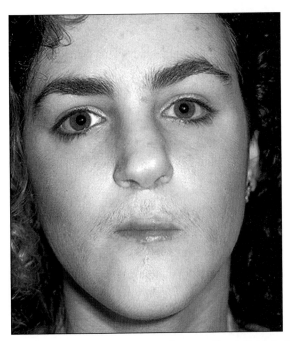

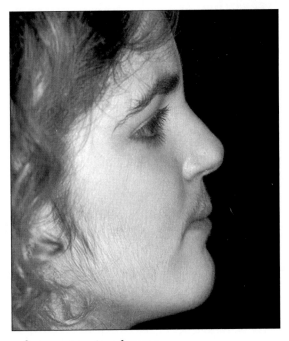

Note the excellent facial changes after surgery to advance the upper jaw and after revision to the nose and lips.

Dental Reconstruction

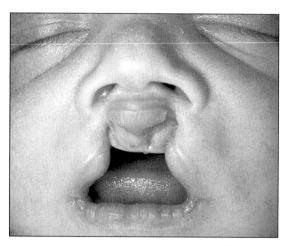

This boy was born with an incomplete bilateral cleft of the lip.

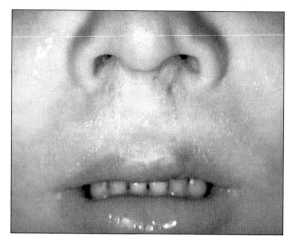

At age 10 years.

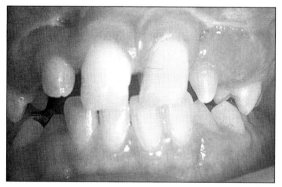

At age 10 years.

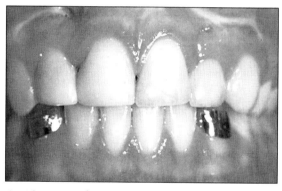

At 12 years of age, his malformed upper front teeth were reconstructed. The upper front teeth were first made more esthetic by the use of composite (bonding) material. The lower band on the teeth held the retainer in place.

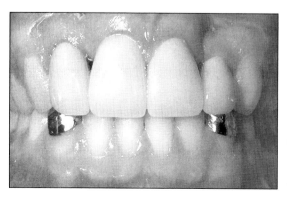

At 16 years of age, porcelain dental laminates (tooth covers) replaced the composite (bonding) material. The bonded lower incisor retainer was removed at 17 years of age.

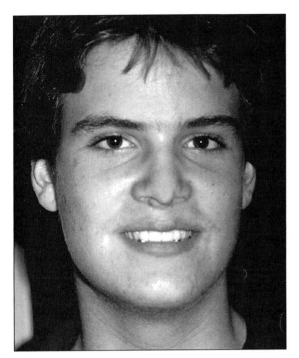 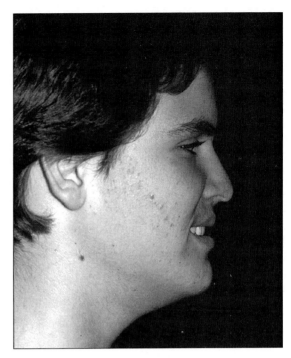

Note the young man's attractive smile and well-developed facial
profile after additional nose and upper lip revisions.

The new upper-to-lower bite relationship is then
recorded in plastic by means of a surgical "wafer" or
index, which will be used by the surgeon as a guide
to properly position the maxillary bony segments.
Metal miniplates are placed over the bone cuts for
stabilization and are usually left in place. When using
intermaxillary fixation (the placement of wires and
elastics between the upper and lower jaws), the surgical wafer is positioned over the teeth and rubber
bands or wires are placed between the upper and
lower jaws for up to six weeks to hold the corrected
dental arches in proper bite relationship while the
bone cuts heal. This method does not permit the
mouth to open. The surgeon or orthodontist will
review proper food preparation should intermaxillary
fixation be necessary.

In some cases, an alternative method (rigid fixation) can be used. This procedure also uses metal

miniplates, which are placed across the bone cuts, to hold the maxillary bony segments in proper position after surgery. However, no wires or rubberbands are placed between the upper and lower jaws. This is more comfortable and allows for normal feeding and speaking even during the healing phase. In some cases, intermaxillary elastics and a surgical wafer may have to be worn for a short period of time even when rigid fixation is utilized.

Before surgery, it may be necessary for the child to donate blood and undergo some laboratory tests at the hospital to be prepared for a possible transfusion. He or she is not to have liquids after midnight the night before surgery. For some procedures, he or she may not need to spend the night before surgery at the hospital, and may even be able to leave the same day.

After orthognathic surgery

Walking as soon as possible after surgery will increase the child's blood circulation, which in turn will help reduce facial swelling. There may be some pain and swelling of the face and neck, most of which should be gone in a couple of weeks. The face itself may feel strange and stiff for a couple of months but will gradually return to normal.

Parents may want to encourage their child to "make faces." Facial grimacing, starting a few days after surgery, can help keep the muscles toned and help reduce swelling.

Hygiene and orthodontic appliances

Keeping the teeth clean after facial skeletal surgery, especially when the jaws are wired together, is difficult but it can and should be done. A soft toothbrush can be used as long as special care is taken not to touch the bruised areas. Food and dental plaque will accumulate on top of orthodontic braces, especially in the areas between the gums and the brackets that are attached to the teeth. To counter this, in addition to careful toothbrushing, a water irrigation device (such as Water Pik) should be used. A vegetable dye (disclosing solution), which can be purchased in a drugstore, will stain any dental plaque left after cleaning to show up areas that need recleaning.

A special diet will be prescribed during this healing period. The orthodontist will tell you which foods your child should avoid when wearing orthodontic appliances. Some examples include hard or sticky substances such as ice, peanuts, caramels, apples, and crunchy, raw vegetables. Such foods can loosen bands and brackets, break arch wires, and promote decay. It is also best to avoid sugar-laden soft drinks, powdered beverages, sweetened juice drinks, cereals with high sugar content, cakes, and pies. Even after the braces are removed, a diet reduced in sugar is recommended.

Other Dental Procedures

These procedures involve replacing missing teeth, or recontouring malformed teeth, to improve facial and dental appearance and speech. Also, in some children with clefts, the treatment is designed to permanently stabilize the palatal segments in their corrected position after orthodontia and orthognathic surgery. When pharyngeal surgery is inappropriate, speech aid appliances may be prepared for controlling air flow between the oral and nasal pharynx. These services are usually performed by a prosthodontist (a dentist specially trained in creating dental prostheses and who has training in treating cleft palate problems) or by a general-practice dentist who also has sufficient experience in this field.

CHAPTER 9

Speech Concerns

The speech defect is the most significant functional disturbance of cleft palate. The production of speech is an acquired skill that initially involves sucking, chewing, swallowing, and breathing. It is an imitative, learned activity that depends on a variety of functioning organs. Since a cleft of the palate prevents the usual bony and muscular separation of the oral and nasal cavities, controlling and directing the air stream during speech become impossible. It is this disturbance that is basic to the speech defect of cleft palate. Cleft lip does not usually result in speech problems.

It is estimated that 10% to 25% of children with clefts of the palate have speech problems resulting from *velopharyngeal insufficiency,* or inadequate closure of the oral-nasal orifice. Other conditions related to clefts can cause problems such as: improper functioning of the muscles that move the soft palate; abnormalities in the size and shape of the muscular and skeletal structures that surround the soft palate due to disturbance in growth; physical interferences with the soft palate function, such as adenoids and tonsils; various types of neuromotor difficulties;

faulty speech learning of unknown origin; and submucous cleft palate. The latter condition can be easily missed; it is characterized by a bifid (split) uvula—that is, there is a cleft in the soft palate and posterior portion of the hard palate masked by intact overlying tissue. Not all children with a submucous cleft have speech problems.

In children with clefts of the palate, surgical repair of the cleft allows for proper feeding, swallowing, and the opportunity to develop normal speech. Without closure of the hard and soft palate, it is sometimes possible for speech to develop normally even without the use of an obturator. However, in most instances, until the palate has been closed, air can escape through the nose, affecting speech sounds. Unable to properly direct speech out of the mouth, children with open clefts may also develop *compensatory* sounds, that is, they may replace speech sounds with abnormal sounds. Such sounds are generally characterized by abnormal tongue and throat movements.

Palate repair alone may not assure ordinary speech development. Although the surgeon may close the palate, the child must still learn to coordinate the sounds of normal speech. Therefore, even after the palate is repaired, some children with clefts will still experience hypernasality (excessive escape of speech sounds through the nose) because of inadequate functioning of the soft palate and/or lateral pharyngeal wall.

In children who also have clefts of the lip and the alveolus with teeth in abnormal positions, articulation (the ability to make specific sounds) may also be impaired. This results from abnormal space in the mouth, the inability to position the tongue tip properly in relation to certain teeth, and an imbalanced relationship between the upper and lower lips.

Finally, chronic hearing loss in early infancy and childhood, due to frequent ear infections (otitis media), may result in impaired acquisition of speech and language skills; that is, without normal hearing ability, a child's speech will be distorted.

Children who have clefts and no other abnormalities should develop language about the same time as other children, and should be encouraged to speak in an uninhibited, natural manner, even if there is excessive nasality and impaired articulation.

Some sounds ordinarily come out of the nose and have a natural nasal resonance, such as *m* and *n*. Therefore, words such as "mama," "no," or "nanny" are generally easier to articulate for the child with a cleft, and they are usually understood by parents without difficulty. Words with sounds that typically do not have any nasal resonance (such as *p, b, t, d, f, v, s,* or *z*) may be difficult for the child to pronounce and for parents to understand—and may therefore go unrecognized.

Difficulty in acquiring normal speech may have negative effects on your child's language development. If sounds cannot be made into words that are understood by others, your child's desire to communicate may be affected. This may delay the development of vocabulary and grammar and sentence construction. If, in your child's case, the onset of speech is late or language acquisition (understanding what is said and expressing oneself) is inadequate, an extensive evaluation should be performed by a speech/language pathologist to determine whether the problem is one of a failure to understand the child's speech, or whether the problem may be related to additional congenital anomalies present in the child.

Your Child's Speech/Language Development

You may have heard that your child's speech may be affected by the cleft and be difficult to understand, but you may not have specific information about the speed of language development. A basic understanding of speech and language development will be of great value to you as your child's verbal abilities begin to develop.

Most children with cleft palate will display the proper speech and language skills for their age, but some will have problems. As parents, you may not know how to approach your child's speech and language development. You may not know what problems might materialize, how to cope with such problems, or what to do to help your child develop normal speech and language skills. The following describes what you can expect regarding your child's speech and language development and how you can play an extremely important role in preventing and correcting possible speech difficulties.

Infancy

Though some cleft palate centers or teams may not suggest contact with a speech/language pathologist until a child reaches his or her third birthday, early stimulation and prevention of problems (between birth and three years of age) is extremely important— this is a child's most important time for speech and language development. If you are given few or no suggestions about hearing, speech, and language stimulation, you are left to conclude that nothing can be done for your child's speech until after surgery. This is not the case! Even at this early age, a multidisciplinary approach is needed in which you are the key component, and the speech/language pathologist, audiologist, pediatrician, and surgeon work together with the family for proper management in the future.

Many cleft palate teams and centers have programs designed to train you in the course of normal speech and language development, how to provide the most enriched speech and language environment for your child, and how to stimulate normal speech development, thus preventing any abnormal speech that may lead to inappropriate sound production by your child. The role of the speech/language pathologist during your child's infant years is to empower you with information so that you and other family members can aid your child's speech and language development. Contact with you and your child soon after birth with continued follow-up to monitor progress and development (every three months until age three) is recommended to provide support and direction to parents, and to allow for therapeutic intervention by the speech/language pathologist as soon as it is judged necessary.

It is important that the speech/language pathologist on the multidisciplinary cleft palate team get to know your child. Frequent contact with him or her can be difficult because of geographical distances, but he or she can coordinate services between the team members and your local speech/language pathologist. The two can work together for the benefit of your child.

What to listen for

Infants begin to produce sounds at two to four months. These sounds (cooing, babbling, and squealing) are initially produced at the back of the mouth and throat and are known as *nonreflexive consonants*. In an infant with a cleft, it is important that the child does not engage in this stage of initial sounds for a prolonged period, because this form of speech has the potential to reinforce inappropriate positioning of the tongue, causing sounds to be made permanently in the back of the mouth and throat. In the normal course of development, nearly all sounds come to be produced in the front of the mouth.

Babbling becomes increasingly elaborate as more complex combinations of sounds are made and the length of the utterances increases. You will want to ensure that the "front of the mouth" sounds *p, b, t,* and *d* are being produced by 14 months.

All sounds are different, so they shouldn't sound the same. Some children with cleft palate may develop a speech pattern that sounds like they are producing *m* or *n* for most of their sounds. Additionally, an increase in the use of sounds not typically heard in your language may alert you to the development of abnormal speech patterns.

The nasal quality (hypernasality) common in children with cleft palates may be very mild or very severe. It is often accompanied by bursts of air (nasal emission) on certain sounds, or there may simply be a general nasal sound (nasal turbulence). A child may exhibit nasal grimacing or unusual facial movements while making certain sounds.

By the age of twelve months, your child should begin to acquire a small vocabulary. By twenty-four months, he or she should be starting to put words together in two-word sentences with a fairly large vocabulary. If these milestones are not reached within two or three months of the expected age, consult a speech/language pathologist. Early parental involvement and the development of positive attitudes toward early speech and language stimulation are extremely important. This calls for parental training—parents must learn those techniques necessary to stimulate normal infant speech development so that the child may achieve normal speech and language function.

What you can do

Accept your child's speech in an atmosphere of warmth and patience. This will provide him or her the best chance to develop normal speech and language. Speak to your child face-to-face so that he or she can see your lips and tongue moving during speech. Exaggerate sounds, making them louder and longer, while using facial expression and inflection in your voice.

Stimulate use of the sounds made at the front of the mouth by using a lot of simple words involving the sounds *p*, *b*, *t*, and *d*, such as "papa," "bye-bye," "top," and "dada." You can do this by talking about what your child is doing and what you are doing, during daily activities such as eating, dressing, bathing, and playing.

You can also have them imitate your labial and dental sounds (*p*, *b*, *t*, and *d*), and reward him or her with attention, smiles, and hugs when these sounds are attempted and made. Engage in sound play with your child using such games as copycat, imitating each other's sounds. You can also engage your child in sound-associated lip and tongue play (making funny faces).

Don't *demand*, however, that your child imitate your correctly produced sounds or words. This will frustrate your child, and you may lose his or her attention. Providing the appropriate sound environment is the key!

Reinforce normal receptive (comprehension) and expressive (verbal) language development by stimulating verbal requests and comments and by increasing your child's vocabulary knowledge and use. Incorporate these recommendations into activities throughout the day, and encourage other family members to use these strategies. Consistency is the key.

If you suspect your infant has a problem in speech and language development, have him or her examined by a speech/language pathologist. Don't wait! It is also important to ensure that your child has adequate hearing by having his or her ears checked by physicians and audiologists. Follow their recommendations. A child needs to *hear* speech sounds for normal speech and language to develop.

Toddlers and School-Age Children

As children approach their third birthday, they should reach certain milestones in their speech and language development. This includes understanding all that is said to them, expressing themselves in one- to three-word sentences, using a vocabulary of approximately one thousand words, and producing most verbal sounds with near accuracy.

By the time a child is twenty-four to thirty months of age, he or she should be producing sounds such as *p, b, t, d, s, f, k,* and *g* fairly clearly. If you suspect your child is having difficulties with articulation (how various sounds are made)—speech is persistently unclear, there is a fair amount of hypernasality, or your child does not sound like others of the same age—a full speech/language evaluation is required.

The Speech/Language Pathologist's Role

The speech/language pathologist will determine your child's speaking ability and distinguish any errors in sounds that may exist. If there are problems with certain sounds, it is important to determine whether these sounds are developmental errors (those that can exist in the speech of any child at a certain age) or errors directly related to the cleft palate.

Along with articulation, the speech/language pathologist will evaluate the amount of air emitted from the mouth and nose (resonance) while your child is speaking. If an excessive amount of air is being emitted from the nose (hypernasality), a determination must be made about whether your child is obtaining adequate closure of the soft palate and side wall muscles (lateral pharyngeal walls) at the opening into the back of the nose (velopharyngeal port). This closure is very important for the production of sound.

Compensatory articulation

If your child is unable to obtain velopharyngeal closure, there may exist a leakage of air through the nose during speech. This may contribute to poor overall understanding of your child's speech by others, and, because of poor muscle "learning," may contribute to your child's use of inappropriate muscles in the throat to produce sounds instead of using the lips and tongue. Such sounds are often regarded as substitutions and you may hear them referred to as "compensatory articulation." The most common compensatory sounds are known as *glottal stops* and *pharyngeal fricatives*. Glottal stops are made with the muscles of the throat (pharynx) and vocal folds (larynx) in an attempt to make the following sounds: *p, b, t, d, k,* and *g.* Glottal stops sound like a grunt, a hard *h,* or a throat sound. Pharyngeal fricatives are sounds that are made at the back of the mouth and throat for *s, z, f, v, sh,* and *ch.* These may sound like a hiss, a lisp, or a friction noise.

The speech/language pathologist will likewise examine the areas of voice, fluency, and language with clinical observation and standardized tests. If there are difficulties in comprehension and expression of language, appropriate recommendations will be made regarding language therapy.

If difficulties in speech production and resonance occur, several clinical studies are required to further diagnose the degree of severity. Videofluoroscopy (an x-ray motion picture of tongue and palate movement during speech) and nasoendoscopy (the use of a fiber-optic scope allowing a direct view of the velopharyngeal muscles during speech) are the two most common diagnostic studies. These studies are usually not performed until the child is four years old and is able to provide an adequate speech sample.

Speech Therapy and Surgical Options

Speech therapy is necessary when your child is producing sounds with distortions or substitutions and when it is difficult to understand more than 20% of what he or she is saying. If a developmental articulation disorder exists, articulation therapy may be recommended. However, if compensatory articulation exists, usually accompanied by hypernasality, the speech pathologist will determine the appropriate course of management in conjunction with rest of the cleft palate team. Several options exist depending on the nature and severity of the compensatory articulation and hypernasality.

With mild-to-severe hypernasality and good oral articulation, several treatment options exist. Some centers and cleft palate teams may suggest a prosthetic obturator to block the cleft space. This acrylic device inserted into the cleft area will stop the air flow into the nose (nasal cavity) and redirect it into the mouth (oral cavity). An alternative is surgical management of velopharyngeal insufficiency. This procedure, often referred to as *pharyngeal flap surgery*, provides a permanent bridge of tissue to limit and direct air flow away from the nose and through the mouth. A pharyngeal flap, which is a sail-like structure, restricts food, liquids, and much of the air from entering the nose. The surgery is a treatment option for hypernasality only; it does not treat articulation problems. An examination performed before surgery helps the surgeon determine what type of flap is required (wide or narrow), the location of the flap, and the direction of the flap (centered or shifted to the right or left). This information ensures greater success in the elimination of hypernasality.

One appliance, the palatal lift appliance, is used in the treatment of palatopharyngeal incompetency only for those cases where the soft palate has been identified as being of inadequate length. Traditionally, palatopharyngeal incompetency has been managed by means of pharyngeal surgery, appliances, or a combination of both. The appliance is recommended when the patient or caregivers do not wish to pursue surgical management. A palatal lift appliance elevates the soft palate with the objective of decreasing the opening of the valve space to normal proportions during speech. Some believe that the appliance improves palatopharyngeal function by constant and continuous stimulation of the soft palate muscle.

The palatal lift appliance may be used from one to four months (continuous or part-time wear) along with articulation therapy. Speech therapy is initiated once the appliance is inserted, and for school-age children the appliance is usually worn only during school hours. A part-time wear schedule can be used on weekends and holidays, or over the summer. It must be stressed that treatment with the palatal lift appliance is not for all patients and is not always successful.

Speech aid appliances can help those with clefts improve their speech.
This appliance carries the speech bulb to the pharynx behind and above the soft palate in order to channel more air through the mouth. The speech bulb (a) fits into the nasopharynx, above the level of the hard palate. The shank (b) carries the speech bulb on one end and is attached to the body of the appliance. The body of the appliance (c) has wire tooth clasps to hold the appliance in place. False teeth may be attached if teeth are missing. It also helps maintain the corrected palatal arch form.

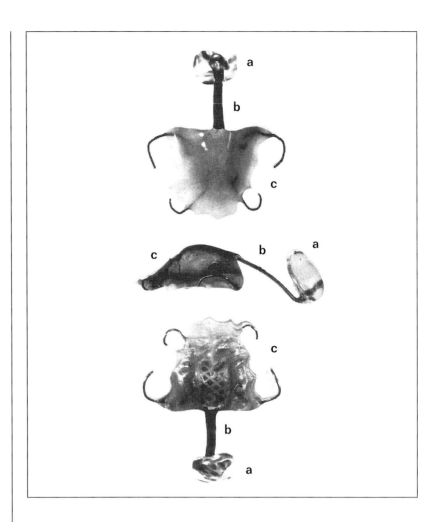

Mild-to-severe hypernasality accompanied by a mild-to-severe compensatory articulation pattern may call for intensive articulation therapy (three to five times per week) to facilitate front-of-the-mouth sounds, air flow through the mouth, and strong sound production. In some cases, intensive articulation therapy may be used in conjunction with a speech bulb appliance. This acrylic bulb on an extended palatal ball-like addition (made by the orthodontist or prosthodontist) fits into the space of the insufficiency. It is used in conjunction with articulation therapy. Some believe it stimulates muscle wall movement, thus reducing the size of the hole.

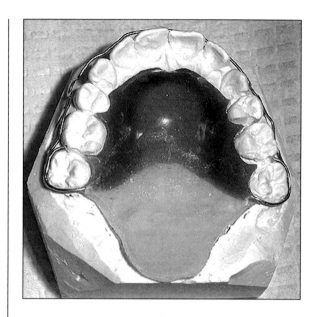

A palatal lift appliance. This appliance is used to elevate the soft palate to improve palatopharyngeal function by continuous stimulation of the soft palate muscle. It is used only when the soft palate is slightly short. The rear extension of the appliance makes contact with the soft palate.

This in turn reduces the hypernasality and, with articulation therapy, facilitates normal sound production. The bulb's size is reduced over time as muscle movement improves. This course of treatment is viable because it can reduce the size of the muscle flap required. This is very important for children with small airways or other congenital anomalies that may affect breathing. Pharyngeal flap surgery may still be an option once the speech bulb reduction program and articulation therapy have been completed (that is, when the maximal potential for velopharyngeal closure will have been achieved).

Speech therapy can be extremely helpful before secondary palatal (pharyngeal flap) surgery. It has been shown to decrease hypernasality, facilitate good front-of-the-mouth articulation, and decrease the complexity of the procedure to be used. At times it eliminates the need for surgery altogether.

Articulation Therapy

Articulation therapy should be structured according to your child's attention span, intellectual and motivational capabilities, and therapeutic needs. Sessions are individualized (one-on-one) and intensive (three to five visits per week) and typically last at least thirty minutes per visit. Parental involvement in the therapeutic process, within the therapy setting as well as in the home, is encouraged as it provides continuity and assures consistency of sound-producing technique. Also, the speech pathologist should be in constant contact with the cleft palate team, as well as with schoolteachers, to update each professional on your child's progress and to discuss future management.

Although many speech pathologists continue to support "muscle training exercises" such as blowing, sucking, and swallowing, such activities *do not* assist in speech production. Good, normal sound production is best facilitated by normal speaking tasks.

Does Orthodontic Therapy Affect Speech?

A highly integrated multidisciplinary team is vital in the care of a child with a cleft because many procedures and treatments may occur at the same time. You may find your child in articulation therapy at the same time orthodontics is being performed. During orthodontic therapy, many appliances are placed in the mouth that may temporarily affect sound production and/or change the tone of the sound (oral resonance). However, that should be of no concern to you at this time.

Braces do not have long-term effects on sound production. Once placed, temporary sound distortions may occur due to displacement of the tongue and lips, but the lips and tongue quickly accommodate the braces and the child easily compensates in speech. If maxillary expansion appliances are used, the place where the tongue contacts the palate for certain sounds may change temporarily. However, the child usually compensates and sounds may be only slightly affected. Maxillary expansion appliances, because they move the palatal segments apart, may expose a small hole (fistula) in the palate. This fistula, which was hidden, may now contribute to hypernasality, decreased air pressure in the mouth, liquids seeping from the nose (nasal regurgitation), or to a compensatory sound pattern. However, fistulas can be temporarily corrected by speech appliances (obturators) or surgically repaired when necessary.

The role of speech/language pathology is an extremely important one in the health care management of your child with a cleft lip and/or palate. Preventing problems in language development is easier than trying to treat them once they are established. The best time to begin preventive measures is during the first few years of life. Keep in mind that a multidisciplinary approach is necessary, one in which you the parent as well as the team members are an integral part of aiding your child's development of normal speech and language skills.

CHAPTER 10

*H*earing Concerns

Infants born with cleft palates and other craniofacial anomalies are likely to have more hearing problems than other infants, and the condition of their middle ear is likely to be of concern for the rest of their lives. Since hearing loss is a major cause of language learning problems, it is important to be on the alert for any signs of hearing impairment in your child. Your child should undergo regular examinations to detect and prevent chronic ear disease and deafness.

The Ear

While hearing is a key factor in communication, possibly even more important is that it gives people a feeling of life participation and security. A sense of hearing is vital to well-being. Anytime there are problems involving the ear, a physician should be consulted.

The normal human ear can distinguish among some four hundred thousand different sounds, some weak enough to cause the eardrum to move as little as one-tenth the diameter of a hydrogen molecule. When a telephone rings, it produces a series of disturbances in the surrounding air, and these disturbances, or sound waves, travel out and away from the source. Your hearing mechanism perceives these and transforms and transmits these sound waves as a message to your brain.

Before the message can get to your brain, however, it has to pass through three well-defined sections of the ear; the outer ear, the middle ear, and the inner ear. The outer ear includes the *pinna*, the part of the ear we can see, plus the ear canal. The pinna is designed to help gather sound waves and funnel them down the ear canal to the eardrum.

The sound waves then strike the eardrum, or *tympanic membrane*, which is about as thin as tissue paper but very strong. The eardrum separates the outer and middle ear. The eardrum vibrates when sound waves strike it. Attached to the eardrum is a chain of three small bones called the *ossicular chain*. The bones are in the pea-sized middle-ear cavity.

The ossicles, the smallest bones in the human body, are full-size when we are born. These individual bones are smaller than grains of rice, and they are named after objects they resemble. The bone attached to the eardrum is the *malleus* (hammer), the second bone is the *incus* (anvil), and the third is the *stapes* (stirrup). As sound waves move the eardrum, they move the ossicles. The three bones actually form a lever system that transfers the energy of the sound waves from the outer ear through the middle ear and into the inner ear.

The *eustachian tube* is the part of the middle ear that connects the middle ear cavity with the back of the throat. The upper end is normally open because it is surrounded by bone. The lower end is normally closed, or collapsed, because it is surrounded by soft tissue. The eustachian tube helps maintain a

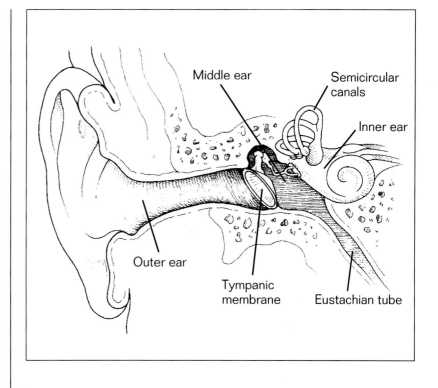

The ear has three chambers: the outer, middle, and inner ear. The two connecting structures are the *semicircular canals* responsible for maintaining balance and the *eustachian tube* for the equalization of air pressure to the middle ear and drainage of fluids to the nose.

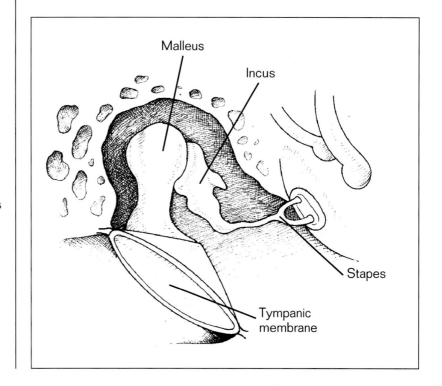

The middle ear contains the *ossicular chain*, which transmits vibrations from the tympanic membrane to the oval window. It is composed of the *malleus, incus,* and the *stapes.* Cleft palates can cause problems with the opening and closing mechanism of the eustachian tube. Malfunction of the eustachian tube can lead to otitis media, inflammation of the middle ear. (Adapted from "Physiology of the Ear," Starkey Laboratories, Inc.)

balance between the air pressure on both sides of the eardrum. The tube opens about every third time we swallow or yawn, allowing air pressure in the middle ear to equalize with the outside air pressure. The normal ear-popping sensation sometimes experienced in an airplane or with other sharp changes in altitude is caused by this equalization process.

The last bone in the ossicular chain, the stapes, is attached to a tiny membrane called the *oval window*. The oval window is an entrance to the inner ear that contains the organ of hearing, or cochlea. When the stapes bone moves, the oval window moves with it. The cochlea is a fluid-filled channel. The fluid is disturbed by movements of the oval window. Inside the cochlea are thousands of microscopic hair-like cells that are set in motion whenever the fluid is disturbed. Stimulation of these cells, in turn, causes electrical impulses to be sent to the brain.

Our inner ears also contain a very important organ that is actually connected to the cochlea but does not contribute to our sense of hearing. Instead, these three small loops, called semicircular canals, help us maintain balance. Problems within the *semicircular canals* may result in symptoms such as dizziness.

Hearing Problems

Individuals with craniofacial anomalies may have congenital abnormalities of the ear structures, and they are thus subject to ear disease. Such children are at high risk for hearing disorders varying from mild to severe. The 1990 Joint Committee on Infant Hearing in the United States recommended that "at risk" newborns have their hearing screened at the age of three months and no later than six months.

Infection of the middle ear is one of the most common problems for all children, and it can be one of the most serious complaints during childhood. An untreated or repeated ear infection can inhibit learning at critical stages of language development because it can reduce a child's ability to hear.

More children with cleft palates suffer decreases in hearing than do similar groups of children without cleft palate. Since it is very difficult to see the eardrum in small infants, the physician and parents may not be initially aware of the presence of ear disease, and changes in the tympanic membrane and bones of the middle ear may occur that might have been prevented by early treatment.

The part of the ear of most concern in the child with a cleft palate is the middle ear. The eustachian tube normally drains fluid that collects during a cold or respiratory infection. The muscles that help the eustachian tube function properly are connected to the soft palate. If there is a cleft palate, these muscles may not operate efficiently, thus interfering with the ability of the eustachian tube to drain fluid from the middle ear to the back of the nose.

A child's eustachian tube is shorter, narrower, and more horizontal than an adult's; for these reasons it is more likely to swell during a cold and become blocked. Poor drainage of the middle ear may lead to the accumulation of fluid (effusion). The effusion may become infected with bacteria or viruses and cause pressure and/or fever. The fluid hampers the movement of the eardrum and associated small bones and may lead to hearing loss. This loss is about the same level of decrease you would get by putting a finger in your ear canal. It is, however, unusual for a child with a cleft palate to experience total hearing loss.

Since these changes occur early in life, the child may not show obvious hearing loss problems but may simply learn to live with the disease. Moderate hearing loss may not be noted until the child is older, when it becomes obvious that he or she does not hear properly. Occasionally, an infection will be severe enough to cause a hole in the eardrum, resulting in a draining ear. While it is difficult to evaluate hearing in infants, it is not impossible. A specialist in the testing of hearing (audiologist) may work with the ear specialist (otolaryngologist or otologist) to evaluate your child's hearing as he or she grows. In almost all children, this team can evaluate the hearing level.

Otitis media

In the later stages of infancy and throughout their childhood, there is a higher incidence of *otitis media,* inflammation of the middle ear, in children with clefts. This suggests a disturbance of some kind around the eustachian orifice. Whether this is caused by an anatomic or functional variation associated with the cleft, or by an increased susceptibility to irritation and infection, remains to be resolved.

Those who suffer from respiratory allergies, as well as infants who usually drink from a bottle while lying down, are at risk for otitis media. Because this disease of the middle ear can cause deafness, prevention and detection are essential.

The basic instrument for examining the ear for otitis media is the otoscope. Another screening technique is tympanometry, which measures the ability of the tympanic membrane to vibrate. Parents should be aware that school screening tests are not always sufficient to identify otitis media.

Management of middle ear disease, elimination of middle ear fluid, and aeration (which balances air pressure between the middle ear and the nasopharynx) of the middle ear are the responsibility of the otologist and can be accomplished by draining (by myringotomy), aspiration (removing fluid by means of suction), or the insertion of tympanotomy or pressure equalization tubes. If the tubes fall out, a myringotomy and reinsertion of the tubes may be necessary. The pressure equalization tubes should be reinserted as many times as necessary until the eustachian tube is functioning adequately. Aeration of the middle ear will prevent serious hearing problems.

Eustachian tube function

The eustachian tube serves three physiologic functions for the middle ear:

1. Ventilation (balancing air pressure between the middle ear and the nasopharynx)
2. Protection (from secretions and pressure)
3. Clearance (draining middle-ear secretions into the nasopharynx)

The normal eustachian tube at rest is closed, with a slight negative pressure existing in the middle ear. There is no muscle tissue in the eustachian tube itself to open or close it. Intermittent contractions during swallowing of the tensor veli palatine muscle, which is attached to the soft palate, cause the eustachian tube to open, equalizing pressure in the middle ear. (This is why repeated swallowing can often relieve painful pressure disequilibrium in the ears during a sharp airplane descent; when the ears "pop," it is a sign that more equalized pressure has been restored.) Yawning and sneezing also open the eustachian tube. Conversely, relaxation of the tensor veli palatine muscle causes the eustachian tube to close.

Obstruction of the eustachian tube may result in a negative pressure in the middle ear. If this persists, atelectasis, or collapse of the tympanic membrane, may occur and lead to the accumulation of fluid in the resulting space. This negative pressure also creates a situation in which bacteria from the nose may be aspirated into the middle ear, resulting in acute bacterial otitis media with effusion.

When a persistent hearing loss is identified, hearing aids and auditory training systems should be considered. When hearing loss occurs in the presence of *atresia* (blockage), whether in one or both ears, bone conduction amplification may be considered. Depending upon degree of loss, an implantable bone conduction aid may be an option in treatment. These treatment programs require continual monitoring. If a child has a hearing loss, the appropriate school official should be notified. If no hearing loss is detected, the child should still have a yearly checkup.

Mechanical obstructions

Mechanical obstructions of the ear, which can adversely affect persons with or without cleft palates, are classified into two types: extrinsic and intrinsic. The extrinsic variety includes obstructions such as cotton swabs, and anatomic abnormalities such as nasal-pharyngeal tumors and enlarged adenoids. Intrinsic obstructions include blockage by secretions resulting from inflammation caused by infection or possibly allergy.

It must be stressed that in children with cleft palate the condition of the middle ear, even with corrective treatment, will remain a concern throughout their lifetime.

How to Prevent Ear Problems

Ear disease can exist with minimal symptoms in all infants. The ears should be examined regularly, and the wax that interferes with seeing the eardrum removed. Hearing tests should be scheduled as early as possible.

When the child with a cleft palate has a cold in the nose, throat, or chest, the ears should be examined to see whether there is an associated ear infection. If there is, it is usually treated with the appropriate antibiotic. When indicated, the eardrum may have to be lanced to allow fluid to escape from the middle ear. Opening the eardrum will not result in bad scars or permanent holes. It may be necessary for your child's surgeon to perform a *myringotomy,* a procedure in which a small slit is made in the eardrum to permit the drainage of trapped fluid. Ventilating tubes may or may not be placed.

If permanent changes in the ears caused by disease can be prevented during infancy, the need for corrective surgery later in life may be avoided. If disease-caused changes do occur, techniques are available to allow the surgeon to try to reconstruct the middle ear in hopes of restoring proper function.

As the child gets older, examining hearing function becomes easier. Periodic hearing tests are valuable throughout childhood and adolescence to determine whether treatment is necessary.

Hearing Tests

Pure-Tone Audiometer. This device provides information about the integrity of the peripheral auditory system, that is, the outer, middle, and inner ear.

Whatever sound-transmitting defect exists in the ear will be revealed on an audiogram as a loss in hearing sensitivity.

Bone-Conduction Audiometry. This procedure basically measures defects of the sensorineural (pertaining to the sensory nerve) mechanism of the ear. The bone-conducted signal bypasses the external and middle ear and goes directly to the inner ear through vibrations of the cranial bones.

The classic method of distinguishing middle ear defects from cochlear or sensorineural impairment is to find the difference between air-conduction and bone-conduction hearing levels (known as the air-bone gap).

Impedance Audiometry. This is an objective hearing test that does not require the child's active participation. This test includes tympanometry, static compliance or acoustic impedance, and acoustic reflex threshold measurements. An instrument is used to detect the possible presence of fluid in the middle ear. The entire battery of three tests can be administered by an experienced person in sixty to ninety seconds per ear. The child can be sedated if necessary, and the tests can be used successfully with persons of all ages, including newborn children.

Tympanometry cannot detect sensorineural hearing impairment and thus cannot be substituted for pure-tone audiometry as a screening technique. However, tympanometry is more sensitive and reliable than air-conduction audiometry in identifying a pathologic condition of the middle ear, and probably is equal or superior in reliability to the otoscopic examination. It is recommended that tympanometry, in combination with air-conduction audiometry, offers the best method for detecting middle ear disease and hearing impairment.

Otoscope. An otoscope is used to visualize the tympanic membrane that separates the middle ear chamber from the outer ear canal. Otologic assessment of the middle ear during the first year of life is important to determine whether or not otitis media is present. Regular examination (every three months) allows prompt treatment if the disease is present.

Audiologic Evaluation Instruments. These hearing evaluation instruments aid in the detection of hearing disabilities. An audiometer, for example, is used to evaluate any degree of hearing loss. The detection of a disability by the physician marks the beginning of a diagnostic process that varies in duration and complexity with the chronological and mental age of the child and the nature of the auditory problem.

CHAPTER 11

What You Need to Know

It's natural for parents to feel that because their child's face is slightly unusual, everything about their child must be different. But that's not so. The child's cleft is only a small part of who he or she is. Instead of focusing on the problem, parents need to focus on the many more things—the countless things—that make their child a wonderful and miraculous gift.

It's a good idea for you as parents to encourage your child to talk about his or her feelings and to be willing to just listen. As the child grows and begins to ask questions, be truthful about the scars; don't blame them on an accident. Even with support and understanding, the older the child becomes, the more "different" he or she will feel, and the youngster may retreat socially. You can help prevent this by providing your child with continuing social and psychological support and by encouraging him or her to not be afraid to enter social situations. Children with visible differences are often ignored, which is one reason that teaching them communication skills is so important.

Psychosocial counseling for you and your child can be most helpful, and you should feel comfortable pursuing it if you feel that it would be beneficial. Remember also that cleft palate team members are ready to answer questions at any stage of your child's treatment; it is important that you understand what is being attempted to reach the goals of good speech, hearing, dental function, and facial appearance. Much will be done to help your child attain these goals, but the process takes time and requires patience and cooperation.

Most of all, keep in mind that a healthy, giving attitude toward your child and toward your spouse—along with realistic expectations about what the cleft palate team can achieve—are of vital importance in rearing a well-adjusted child who just happens to have a cleft.

Bill of Rights and Responsibilities for Patients and Parents

It is important for you to know what your child's rights are as a patient and what your rights and obligations are as a parent and client of the hospital. Some hospitals have adopted a set of written principles to help ensure that your child receives appropriate medical care. Talk with those involved in your child's care. What follows are the guiding principles of patient care adopted by Miami Children's Hospital.

You and your child have the right

1. To considerate, respectful care and to privacy consistent with the care prescribed. This includes consideration of the psychosocial, spiritual, and cultural variables that influence the perceptions of illness.

2. To know by name the physicians, nurses and staff members responsible for your child's care; to receive responses to questions and requests; and, to receive information regarding your child's diagnosis, the treatment prescribed, the prognosis of the illness, and any instruction required for follow-up care, in language you understand.

3. To know what patient support services are available to you and your child.

4. To request a consultation or second opinion from another physician; to change physicians; to change hospitals.

5. To participate in decisions regarding the medical care of your child. To the extent permitted by law, this includes the right to refuse consent for treatment; to cross out and initial any part of a consent form that you do not want applied to your child's care; to withdraw consent, and to be informed of the consequences of these actions.

6. To participate in the consideration of ethical issues arising in the care of your child through the Hospital Bioethics Committee.

7. To expect all communications and other records pertaining to your child's care, including the source of payment for treatment, to be kept confidential except as needed for proper treatment and hospital administration, or as authorized by appropriate consent, or otherwise provided by law or third-party payment contract.

8. To be informed of the hospital's policies regarding payment; to request, prior to treatment, an estimate of charges for medical care; and to request information and counseling on the availability of known financial resources for your child's care.

9. To receive an itemized bill, and to request an explanation of the charges.

10. To have access to the medical resources of the hospital indicated for your child's care without regard to race, national origin, religion, handicap, or source of payment.

11. To treatment for emergency medical conditions that will deteriorate from failure to receive treatment.

12. To information about medical treatment given for the purpose of research, or research being conducted in addition to medical treatment; and, to refuse to participate in research, with the assurance that care will not be adversely affected by such a refusal.

13. To express concerns or complaints regarding these rights or the quality of care and service provided by the hospital to the Department of Patient/Family Relations.

You have the responsibility

1. To know and follow the rules and regulations of the hospital and the particular unit. Parents or other responsible adults should accompany minor children on any hospital visit and observe all hospital rules.

2. To provide, to the best of your knowledge, accurate and complete information about present complaints, past illnesses, hospitalizations and other matters relating to your child's health; and, to report unexpected changes in your child's condition.

3. To notify your child's physician or nurse if you do not

understand a diagnosis, treatment or prognosis; and, to ask for clarification if you do not understand papers you are asked to sign.

4. To cooperate and to follow the care prescribed or recommended for your child by the physician, nurses or allied health personnel.

5. To keep your appointments and to be on time. When an appointment cannot be kept, the hospital or the clinic should be notified as soon as possible to cancel the appointment and arrange for a new one.

6. For your actions and their consequences if you refuse treatment for your child, or do not follow the physician's instructions.

7. To assure that the financial obligations associated with your child's care are fulfilled as promptly as possible.

8. To be considerate of the rights of other patients and hospital personnel by assisting in the control of noise, the number of visitors your child receives, and by observing the no-smoking policy. Note: you are welcome to stay in your child's room provided the rules and regulations are adhered to. Exception: Parents of patients in the intensive care units and in the psychiatric inpatient unit are not permitted to stay in the room with their child.

9. To advise your nurse, physician, or any members of your health care team of any dissatisfaction you may have with your child's care.

The Department of Patient/Family Relations is responsible for pursuing any questions, concerns, or formal complaints you may have about your rights or the quality of care and service provided by your hospital. You may contact the departmental staff directly, or ask any staff member to contact them on your behalf. Your complaint will not adversely affect your child's care and the staff will welcome the opportunity to address your concerns and be of assistance.

*F*inancial Assistance and Other Resources

Financial resources to help in paying all or part of the costs of treating a person with a cleft lip and/or palate fall into three general categories: private and group health insurance; federal and state resources; and private and nonprofit agencies, foundations, and local service organizations. The most important thing to remember is that there are funds available, and people available, to help the person with a cleft get the care he or she needs.

Health Insurance

Private and group health insurance will usually cover a portion of the cost of treatment of a cleft lip or palate after a deductible is met. Check your health-care plan or call your insurance company for specific coverage information. When choosing health insurance policies, check into coverage of not only surgery and medical care but also dental care and services such as hearing testing, speech and language testing and treatment, and psychological testing and/or counseling. If you are being denied the coverage benefits set forth in your policy, call and advise your State Insurance Board.

Seeking Insurance from Private Companies

Without the active and thorough involvement of parents in the claims process, insurance companies do not always fulfill their contractual obligations in a complete or timely way. "Insurance Issues," an article written by Teresa Robinson that appeared in *About-Face*, August/September 1992, says it all.

Seventeen years ago, on the day my son was born, I had no idea how much my life would change. A child with special needs takes an incredible amount of energy, time, care, and last, but not least, money!

Eric was born with a bilateral cleft lip and palate. Through his 28 surgeries, I have dealt with the insurance company on almost every claim. The first few surgeries were covered by Crippled Children's Services (now usually called Children's Special Health Services [CSHS] in most states) because my husband was in school and we had very little income. I had checked with other service organizations, but was unable to receive any assistance. Since 1985, I have kept accurate records. The insurance companies have disputed almost every claim. The following are but a few examples of conditions related directly to his birth defect that we have had to seek legal counsel to get resolved.

Eric needed a hearing aid. The insurance company claimed that they would only pay for this if Eric had been in an accident and the hearing aid was intended to restore his hearing, not to give him hearing.

Eric had speech therapy for ten years. The same rules held for this therapy as for the hearing aid, and the insurance company would not provide for speech therapy, regardless if it was due to his birth defect or not.

Eric has needed braces and other orthodontic appliances. The dental insurance has paid for some, but Eric has now reached the coverage limit. The medical insurance refuses to pay. This orthodontic battle is now before the city's legal department. The latest orthodontic work is in preparation for upcoming surgery and is a necessary step before this can occur. The insurance company states that treatment is orthodontic and denies coverage.

Presently, I deal with a self-insured employer. My motto has become "Don't accept no for an answer." After the first denial, I would write to the broker again, enclosing a doctor's letter. If coverage is still denied, I suggest going directly to the employer, who can overrule the broker. If all else fails, see an attorney. Each claim dispute can take anywhere from six months to two years to be processed.

Federal and State Government Resources

Medicaid

Medicaid (Title XIX of the Social Security Act of 1966) is a federal assistance program that covers most of the cost of medical care for people with low incomes who require hospital or physician services or certain laboratory and x-ray procedures. In some states, services such as treatment for speech or hearing defects may be covered. Apply in the county offices of your state Social Service, Welfare, or Human Resources Departments.

Children's Special Health Services (CSHS)

Formerly called the Crippled Children's Program, CSHS provides comprehensive medical care to children under the age of 21 who have congenital or acquired physically handicapping conditions. Specific medical and financial criteria have to be met by the applicants before financial assistance is approved. Applications are available through the director of Children's Special Health Services. Contact your state Department of Health for further information or for the locations of agencies or medical facilities in your community that provide these services.

Vocational Rehabilitation Services

These services are designed for persons sixteen years of age or older with emotional, mental, physical/medical, and/or developmental disabilities that hinder their prospects for employment. Call your state Department of Human Resources or Welfare Office for assistance in locating the nearest VR services.

Champus

Champus is a federally funded medical benefits program for members of the uniformed services and their dependents. For more information, contact the health benefits administrator at the nearest military installation.

The Federal Hill-Burton Act

These funds provide for indigent care at hospitals for which federal monies were used for construction. Your hospital's admissions office will have information on the availability of these funds and guidelines for eligibility.

Public Law 99-457

This law better enables parents to secure services for their children younger than two years of age who have identifiable handicaps. The law is scheduled to be in full operation by 1994. Each state has developed its own implementation plan. For more information, contact your state's Education Department or Department of Health and Rehabilitative Services.

US Department of Health and Human Services, Maternal and Child Health Bureau, The Program for Children with Special Health Care Needs

To participate in this program, public schools must offer an assessment and a written Individualized Family Service Plan (IFSP) for the child and parents. Educational services may include: special education, speech and language pathology, audiology, psychological services, parent training, and medical services for diagnostic purposes to enable the child to benefit from early intervention. For more information, write to: US Department of Health and Human Services, Maternal and Child Health Bureau, 5600 Fisher Ln, Rockville, MD 20857.

Private and Nonprofit Agencies, Foundations, Service Organizations, and Support Groups

The Association for the Care of Children's Health

This organization is devoted to improving ways in which the health-care community responds to the unique emotional and developmental needs of children. It sponsors a Parent Network for parents of children with special needs. This network seeks, among other things, to increase awareness of the availability of services and resources at the local, state/province, and national level and to develop methods for receiving and disseminating the most current information. It also seeks to strengthen the skills of parents in initiating parent-to-parent outreach, and to promote the inclusion of families who have traditionally not been well-served by the health-care system because of race, culture, ethnicity, socioeconomic status, or the nature of their children's illness. For more information, contact ACCH, 7910 Woodmont Ave, Ste 300, Bethseda, MD 20814-3015, (301) 654-6549.

The Alliance of Genetic Support Groups

For information, write: The Alliance of Genetic Support Groups, 35 Wisconsin Circle, Ste 440, Chevy Chase, MD 20815

The Cleft Palate Foundation

This foundation is the fundraising, educational, and communication component of the American Cleft Palate Craniofacial Association, providing free information for parents and patients about such topics of interest as local treatment facilities and parent support groups. For more information, write: The Cleft Palate Foundation, 1218 Grandview Ave, Pittsburgh, PA 15211; or call (412) 481-1376 or 1-800-24-CLEFT. (See Appendix D for publications.)

The Miami Craniofacial Anomalies Foundation

The MCAF supports research and education in cleft palate and other craniofacial malformations. Donations may be sent to: The Miami Craniofacial Foundation, 6601 SW 80th St, South Miami, FL 33143; or call (305) 667-3126 for more information.

The National Association for the Craniofacially Handicapped (FACES)

FACES provides financial assistance for supportive services, eg, transportation, food, and lodging to families of individuals who are receiving treatment for craniofacial deformities resulting from birth defects, injuries, or disease. For further information write to: FACES, PO Box 11082, Chattanooga, TN 37401; or call (615) 266-1632.

The Easter Seal Society

Easter Seal is a nonprofit organization serving physically or developmentally disabled children and adults. Although the Society's primary focus is on patients with cerebral palsy and similar neurologic conditions, local chapters provide a variety of other services including speech and hearing assistance. For a description of Easter Seal services in your area, contact your state office or write: The National Easter Seal Society, 2023 W Ogden Ave, Chicago, IL 60612. (See Appendix D for publications.)

Grottos of America

Grottos of America provides dentistry to the handicapped. Patients must be under eighteen years of age to receive assistance from this organization. In addition they must have one of the following conditions: cerebral palsy, muscular dystrophy, mental retardation, or myasthenia gravis. For further information about the organization's national headquarters, write: Grottos of America, 1696 Brice Rd, Reynoldsburg, OH 43068; or call (614) 860-9193.

La Leche League International

La Leche League, a society consisting of lay and professional members, provides accurate information and a variety of support services to parents and health-care professionals committed to breast feeding. For more information write: La Leche League International, 9616 Minneapolis Ave, Franklin Park, IL 60131; or call (708) 455-7730.

The March of Dimes Birth Defect Foundation

The March of Dimes supports programs designed to prevent birth defects and promotes research, professional education, and treatment. Each local chapter determines how its local funds are to be allocated. While chapters are not encouraged to use funds for the treatment of individuals, a local chapter may assist families in meeting the costs of treatment when no other funds are available. Local chapters of the March of Dimes are listed in the telephone directory. For more information write: The March of Dimes, 1275 Mamaroneck Ave, White Plains, NY 10605. (See Appendix D for publications.)

The Natural Father's Network

This organization advocates for fathers of children with disabilities. For more information write: The Natural Father's Network, Merrywood School, 16120 NE Eighth St, Bellevue, WA 98008; or call (206) 282-1334.

Parent Training Information Projects (PTI)

Each state has a PTI office. By contacting a regional office, parents of children with special needs can get information and training and can network with others in their state. To get the phone number of your state office, contact: The Federation for Children with Special Needs, (617) 482-2915, and ask for the CAPP (Collaboration Among Parents and Health Professionals) project; or write: FCSN, 95 Berkeley St, Boston, MA 02116.

Local Service Organizations

The Lions, Sertoma, Kiwanis, and Civitan Clubs sometimes provide emergency one-time financial aid to community members in need if funds are available. Local churches and church-related groups, such as the Knights of Columbus and Masons, may also serve as resources. Telephone numbers for these organizations can usually be found in the Yellow Pages under the heading, "Clubs, Fraternal Organizations, and Religious Organizations."

Health-Care Financing News

Bibliography on Health-Care Financing

To request a copy, write: Collaboration Among Parents and Health Professionals (CAPP), Federation for Children with Special Needs, 95 Berkeley St, Boston, MA 02116; or phone (617) 482-2915.

Health Insurance Resource Guide

The Alliance of Genetic Support Groups has recently published a booklet on understanding the language of health insurance in plain English. Contents include: "The Pre-Existing Condition Dilemma," "Obtaining and Keeping Health Insurance," "Listings of States with High Risk Insurance Pools," "Sample Letters to Contest Insurance Company Decisions," and "Health Insurance in Foreign Countries." For more information about health insurance, or to obtain a copy of this booklet, contact: Martha Volner, AGSG, 1001 22nd St, NW, Ste 800, Washington, DC 20037; or call 1-800-336-GENE.

New Legislation in California Mandating Insurance

New legislation recently passed in California mandates that insurance companies provide continuous hospital, medical, and surgical coverage for the care of children with congenital deformities, including those whose families transfer coverage to another third-party payer. The law was signed by Governor Pete Wilson and specifically targets private insurance companies that claim these anomalies are pre-existing conditions. In the past, if parents switched jobs or changed carriers they risked losing coverage, an all too grimly familiar story. Similar legislative plans exist in Louisiana, Colorado, and Minnesota.

SSI Benefit Denials Under Review

Nearly one-half million children with disabilities who were denied Supplemental Security Income (SSI) benefits during the last ten years are eligible for reevaluation of their claims as a result of the US Supreme Court's recent ruling in Sullivan v. Zebley. Parents and guardians of children with disabilities who were denied benefits, or whose benefits were terminated between January 1, 1980, and February 27, 1990, were sent letters in July 1991 explaining their eligibility for review. Those who have not received a letter, but believe they are eligible, should contact their local Social Security offices.

*T*ips on Financing Health Care*

Families who are finding it harder and harder to obtain or keep adequate health benefits for their children need immediate help with this complex process. They need information and answers to a variety of questions. As families learn more about how the health financing system works, they are often able to help other families do the same.

Read whatever you can find about your child's special health condition. Written materials may mention new equipment, services, or supplies that you want to research further. Ask your child's health-care providers for suggested reading material. Newsletters from self-help organizations and advocacy groups often offer additional helpful information.

Adapted from Paying the Bills: Tips for Families on Financing Health Care for Children with Special Needs, a booklet prepared by parents to share information and strategies for getting health-care payment for children with special needs. Contributors: Eleanora Wells, Maureen Mitchell, Holly Cole, Terry Ohlson, Cheryl Gresek, and Marion Wachtenheim; with special assistance from: Susan G. Epstein, Alexa S. Halberg, and Ann B. Taylor; in collaboration with: New England SERVE Regional Task Force on Health Care Financing, which is supported by a grant through the Maternal and Child Health Bureau, Department of Health and Human Services.

A copy of the booklet may be obtained from New England SERVE, 101 Tremont St, Ste 812, Boston, MA 02108; or call (617) 574- 9493.

Talk to other parents, both individually and through parent groups. Let your child's doctors or other professionals know of your willingness to talk with other parents. Parent meetings or support groups may also offer you new and/or specific information about useful services or equipment and how to obtain them.

Insurance Plans

Traditional Indemnity Plans

These used to be the most familiar type of insurance plans. The insurance company covers some percentage of the cost of the service, with the remaining cost being the responsibility of the family. While traditional indemnity plans allow you the widest choice of providers, your out-of-pocket costs may be higher than some other plans require.

Managed Care Plans

There are now many alternatives to traditional indemnity plans. Managed care plans such as health maintenance organizations (HMOs) and preferred provider organizations (PPOs) contract with providers to deliver health care to a group or individual for a preset fee. A major difference between these types of plans and the traditional indemnity plans is that your choice of providers may be restricted. It is important, therefore, to check on whether the plan includes providers you want to use for your child's specific needs.

Most people purchase their health insurance through their employer and are therefore part of a group plan. These plans usually provide you with the best coverage for the least cost because the risks are being spread over a group. Self-employed people may be able to join a group health plan offered by a professional, trade, or fraternal organization, an association of small businesses, a chamber of commerce, or another group.

The applicant will be asked to provide information about present and past medical history and must agree to release medical records. This may mean that pre-existing conditions will not be covered for a period of time, if at all. In some cases, you may not be able to buy coverage because of a pre-existing condition. In some states, Blue Cross/Blue Shield is required to offer individual health insurance policies, regardless of preexisting conditions. These nongroup plans tend to be costly, offer limited benefits, and may require a waiting period for covering pre-existing conditions.

Check any plan to see what provisions it has for renewal. A renewal process may result in changes in your premiums or benefits.

Insurance companies and managed care plans are businesses, and you and the company you work for are the consumer. They have sold you a product and you should expect the best quality as well as courteous and helpful service.

Most of your communication with the insurer will be by phone. When you contact the insurer, ask for an "800" telephone number, which will save you money. If no toll-free number is available, ask the insurer to call you back. Have a list of specific questions ready for each phone call and take notes on what was discussed. Keep careful records of who you talk to; write down the date, the person's name, position, and telephone number, and take brief notes on what was discussed.

Public Assistance Programs

There are a variety of public programs in every state that might provide health-care benefits to your child with special needs. Although some of these programs are partially funded by the federal government, such as Medicaid, Programs for Children with Special Health Care Needs, Early Interventions, and Special Education, the eligibility requirements and benefits offered will vary state by state. In addition, there may be special programs that your state has developed for children with special health needs or for uninsured or high-risk individuals.

You will need to investigate each program within your state to find out what specific services may be available for your child. The Program for Children with Special Health Care Needs, which is funded through the Maternal and Child Health (MCH) Block Grant in your state, is a good starting place. These programs are mandated to be a source of information and referral, and have a statewide toll-free "800" number.

Ask for a written list of benefits including any restrictions on the amount of these benefits and a description of eligibility criteria. Ask about the application process, any supporting data you will need to supply in your application, and when this information will need to be updated after your initial application.

Ask for help in seeking out and coordinating all possible sources of funding. If your child is covered by a variety of payors, both public and private, request a meeting. Ask all payors to sit down with you and your child's providers, if possible, to map out a financing plan. This is an opportunity for you to have an active role in planning and coordinating your child's care. If your state has a case management or care coordination program for which your child is eligible, the case manager may help to bring this group together.

Organizing Multisource Benefits and Bills

Your child's medical bills may be confusing for several reasons. Billing procedures vary. In some cases, providers require that you pay them directly and then submit a claim to your insurer for reimbursement. In other cases, the provider will bill the insurer directly and you are billed any amount left unpaid. You may be billed by several providers or departments for the same procedure or hospital stay. For example, you may receive a bill from a hospital or medical facility for a test or procedure, a separate bill from the physician who reads or interprets the test, and another bill from the physician who is in charge of your child's care. Many parts of the bill and your insurance company's explanation of benefits may be written in code and therefore may be confusing. Although it is hard to keep track of all this paperwork, it is important to have an accurate record in order to avoid later hassles. Whenever you have questions, ask for clarification.

Keep all information about your child's coverage handy, including policy or identification numbers, billing addresses, and telephone numbers. Keep a copy of each bill you receive and each claim form you have submitted for your files. You may need these copies if any questions arise. Filing these by date of service and keeping insurance forms and provider bills together will help. Staple bills to claim forms when submitting.

Providers may have prearranged billing agreements with different payors. Be sure to let providers know at the time of each service who your possible payors are, including all up-to-date identifying information. Ask for help and cooperation from the providers in order to coordinate your benefits and get the most coverage for a particular service. Give providers any referral forms or signed claim forms that your plan requires at the time of service.

Bills should include dates of service and full descriptions for charges. Bills will probably be sent out to you monthly, but only the first copy sent may have the complete billing information. Therefore, subsequent bills may be confusing. There are special code numbers for each procedure or service. Reimbursement is sometimes denied because this information (dates, descriptions, codes) is incomplete. Look at each bill carefully as soon as you get it. Call the provider for clarification if any information is unclear or inaccurate. In addition, request that your provider send you copies of all bills sent directly to your insurer for payment.

Keep track of bills that have been paid. Your insurance company will send you an estimate of benefits (EOB) or statement of benefits paid or denied. Public programs may not send you these statements, however, unless you request them. Match these statements to your provider bills to track what has been paid, to report any errors, and to keep track of balances due. This may require some detective work, especially if the insurer has lumped several claims together. Sorting out what has been paid will enable you to know what remaining charges are your responsibility and what the insurer still owes. Call the insurance company if you have any questions.

Get Acquainted with Your Insurance Representatives

There is always a chain of command for decision-making about claims. If you are part of a group plan, start by identifying the person who negotiates the health benefits for the group, as well as the representative within the insurance company who is assigned to your group plan. Let them know about your child's specific needs. If you have purchased an individual plan, the agent who sold you the policy and the representative within the insurance company may be helpful if they know your needs.

Try to talk with the same person each time you call so that he or she can get to know you and your child's needs. Complicated questions or requests may need to be answered by another level of decision-maker. Always ask the person you are talking to you if he or she is able to make the decision, and if not, who you should talk to. Remember to keep records of your conversation.

Request statements, promises, or decisions in writing or offer to send a letter with your understanding of the discussion. Keep a copy of your letter. Ask for the date by which you can expect a specific action, payment, or written response. Call back if you do not get a response. Do not easily accept "no" for an answer. "No" really means ask someone else!

Emergency Care Coverage

In order for you to receive payment for certain services, equipment, or scheduled hospitalization, many public and private programs require that you request prior approval. Most plans require notification within 24 hours of any emergency hospitalization. You need to know when prior approval is necessary, how it is to be requested, and any rules for notifying the plan or program for services to be covered. Always ask for a copy of the approval in writing.

Getting the Most from Multisource Insurance

Your child may be covered by more than one health plan. For example, when each parent has a benefit plan through work, or when a child has both insurance and public benefit, there will be multiple payors. Each agency may want to be the payor of "last resort." Try to clarify who will pay for what by asking directly. If an insurer or public program indicates that they think your request may be denied, ask if they could fund part of your request. Another strategy is to ask, "Who do you think should pay for this need?" If all else fails, ask for the name of the supervisor of the person to whom you are talking and start over.

You must describe the medical necessity of the service or equipment that you are requesting for your child. For example, if your child needs special formula or diet supplements, have your doctor write a prescription for the product to demonstrate the medical necessity. Make it clear that any supplies or equipment are intended solely for use by your child for treatment of a medical problem. Use the right language. Avoid words such as "respite," "educational," or "custodial care" with insurance companies or many Medicaid programs. These terms often trigger a rejection of your claim. Use medical terms and concepts such as "home nursing" and "therapeutic services" instead.

Explain how the service or equipment will prevent more costly medical needs in the future. For example, if adequate speech therapy for a child will prevent costly hospitalization and surgery, say so. Cost savings is a very effective rationale for getting approval to pay for services or equipment.

It helps to have identified some key allies among your child's providers who can help you to document your case. The clinic coordinator and/or director may also have good ideas about what should be included in the documentation or request. Ask them to help you describe why the service or equipment is medically necessary.

How to Appeal Claim Denials

Either private plans or public programs may deny your application for benefits. Don't be surprised. Insurance companies are usually not penalized when they deny a claim, even if they are later found to be responsible. Public programs such as Medicaid also deny some claims, which are later accepted. Do not be discouraged by an initial negative response.

Always ask why a claim was rejected, and request this explanation in writing. It may be because the documentation was incomplete or even inaccurate. It may be due to the wording of a request. Sometimes, just by sheer persistence, you can get a company or a program to rethink a decision.

Keep complete records so that you are always ready to resubmit your claim. New procedures or treatments may require insurance companies and public programs to develop new policies. An initial rejection may be due to the insurer's lack of experience with a particular service or equipment. Be understanding, but persistent. All companies and programs make exceptions, so ask for one. Decisions are sometimes made on a case-by-case basis. Be sure to ask that all exceptions, when agreed upon, are put in writing.

All public programs will have a process for appealing decisions. Ask for their policy in writing and for assistance in filing an appeal. Every private plan should also have an appeals process. Ask the insurance company or HMO for a written copy of their policy regarding appeals. The insurance agent who sold you a private policy may be willing to help you negotiate with the insurance company. Your state Insurance Commissioner will have the regulations for and information about the appeals process in your state. This agency may also be helpful to you in appealing your claim. Redocument your child's medical need for the service or equipment. Include letters from professionals such as physicians, therapists, and teachers explaining the importance of this medical need when you resubmit your claim.

If you feel that your request has been wrongfully denied, you may want to seek the advice of a lawyer.

A lawyer might be able to assist you in interpreting your policy or evaluating your disagreement with the insurer or program. Do not reject this possibility because you feel it may be too expensive. There are groups in every state that offer free legal services to families who meet financial eligibility guidelines. Contact a disability advocacy group to help you locate the Legal Services Office or a protection and advocacy agency in your state. These are two publicly funded programs offering professional legal advice. These agencies may also be able to offer some guidance over the telephone regardless of your income. Your state Bar Association may maintain a list of attorneys who do pro bono work and who may be willing to donate their time to help you. You can also ask your employer or union if there is a legal representative available to assist you.

If you disagree with a decision made by a private insurer or HMO on either a claim or application, file a formal complaint with the Commissioner of Insurance in your state. He or she may be able to investigate the issues in your complaint, and at the very least, your complaint provides important evidence of unmet needs. If you are covered by a public program and your appeal is denied, you will want to write letters documenting your need and their denial to the director of the program, the funding source of the program, and your legislators. Names and addresses of legislators are available at your local library. Legislators need to know how public programs are serving their constituents. A single letter with copies sent to the others is fine.

Further Readings

Some of these books may be available from a local parent resource center or your public library.

Fighting Back Health Insurance Denials

Robert Peterson, JD, with David Tenenbaum, MA

This practical guide introduces parents of children with special needs to the world of health insurance. The authors outline the most common reasons that claims are denied and include tips for getting the best type of coverage, strategies for combatting claim denials, arguments and evidence parents can present to insurance companies, and, finally, what to do when all else fails. $14.95. Published by the Center for Public Representation, Inc, 121 S Pickney St, Madison, WI, 53703. Orders may be placed by calling 1-608-251-4008.

Health Insurance Made Easy . . . Finally: How to Understand Your Health Insurance So You Start Saving Your Money and Stop Wasting Your Time

Sharon L. Stark

This manual for consumers written by a former health insurance company employee includes specific information on understanding your health insurance policy and how to submit claims. 1989, 100 pp. $14.95 plus $2.00 postage and handling. To order, write: Stark Publishing, PO Box 8693, Shawnee Mission, KS 66208.

Strategic Insurance Negotiation: An Introduction to Basic Skills for Families and Community Mental Health Workers

Kathy M. Neville

This brief pamphlet, written by a lawyer, offers suggestions to help families negotiate with insurance companies. 1991, 7 pp. Single copies free. To order, write: CAPP/NPRC Project, Federation for Children with Special Needs, 95 Berkeley St, Ste 104, Boston, MA 02116.

Resources for People with Facial Differences

Organizations

AboutFace

AboutFace is an international information and support organization for people with facial differences and their families. Their resources include parent support training, books, videos, and a lending library. (See Appendix D for publications.) AboutFace holds training workshops for people interested in giving school presentations and for those who would like to participate in the support-person visitation program. Other resources include a Cleft Care Kit for parents and professionals, and *Making the Difference,* an orientation package for health-care providers working with a newborn. The National Cleft Palate Association became part of AboutFace in the spring of 1992, and new chapters are being developed throughout North America. Membership, at $20 per year, includes a bimonthly newsletter. For more information, write: Pam Onyx, AboutFace, 1002 Liberty Ln, Warrington, PA 18976; 1-800-225-FACE; FAX (215) 491-0603; or in Canada, contact:

Betty Bednar, AboutFace, 99 Crown's Ln, Toronto, Ontario, Canada M5R 3P4; or call (416) 944-3223; FAX (416) 944-2488.

American Cleft Palate Craniofacial Association (ACPCA) and Cleft Palate Foundation (CPF)

The ACPCA is a professional organization that includes twenty-seven different disciplines. It offers conferences, medical journals, booklets, and other benefits. Membership is open to qualified individuals involved in treatment or research of cleft lip, cleft palate, and other craniofacial anomalies.

The CPF is the fundraising, educational, and communication component of the ACPCA, providing free information for parents and patients. The CPF has a newsletter ($7.50 per year) and a CLEFTLINE for parents of newborns (1-800-24-CLEFT). (See Appendix D for publications.) For more information, write: ACPCA, Nancy Smythe, 1218 Grandview Ave, Pittsburgh, PA 15211; or call (412) 481-1376.

Association for the Care of Children's Health

ACCH, an international organization for health-care professionals and parents, is on the forefront of making medical settings into places where children and their loved ones can best heal and deal with illness. A free newsletter for parents, *ACCH Network,* is available. Their publications include such booklets as *Preparing Your Child for Repeated Hospitalizations; Guidelines for Developing Community Networks; Chronic Illness and Handicapping Conditions: Meeting the Needs of Children and Families; Organizing and Maintaining Support Groups for Parents of Children with Chronic Illness and Handicapping Conditions; and Television and the Hospitalized Child: Issues and*

Creative Approaches. A resource catalog lists films, videos, books, and bibliographies related to special health-care needs, death and bereavement, family education, psychosocial programming in hospitals, and pediatric health-care delivery. A quarterly professional journal, which comes with membership, publishes research studies, essays, and letters. Annual parent and professional meetings are also offered; parents may apply for stipends to attend the annual conference. For more information, write: The Association for the Care of Children's Health, 7910 Woodmont Ave, Ste 300, Bethesda, MD 20814; or call (301) 654-6549.

F.A.C.E.

The Friends for Aid, Correction, and Education of Craniofacial Disorders raises money and gives support to people who need reconstructive surgery. For further information, write: Bernice Bergen, PO Box 1424, Sarasota, FL 34230; or call (813) 955-9250.

Face to Face

Formed by Julie Breuninger, a nurse and the mother of a child with Crouzon's Syndrome, this organization offers phone consultations for parents, as well as area meetings. For an article about parenting a child with Crouzon's written by Ms. Breuninger, write to: Julie Breuninger, 473 Live Oak Dr, El Cajon, CA 92020.

FACES

The National Association for the Craniofacially Handicapped assists people with craniofacial deformities resulting from birth defects, injuries, or disease. Eligible candidates may apply to this nonprofit organization for financial assistance for nonmedical costs. Support is offered on the basis of financial and medical need for such expenses as travel, lodging, and food when traveling to a craniofacial center for reconstructive surgery. To contact FACES for quarterly newsletter, information about craniofacial disorders, support networks, and/or applications for financial assistance, write: FACES, Box 11082, Chattanooga, TN 37401; or call (615) 266-1632.

Federation for Children with Special Needs

The federation is the main headquarters of a national network of parent information centers. Activities include the CAPP National Resource Center for Children with Special Healthcare Needs. The federation is also a coalition of parent-run organizations for children with a variety of disabilities within Massachusetts. Newsletters, workshops, and information sheets are available by writing: The Federation for Children with Special Needs, 95 Berkeley St, Ste 104, Boston, MA 02116-3104; or call (617) 482-2915 (voice or TDD); or toll-free 1-800-331-0688.

Forward Face

A parent-to-parent support organization associated with the Institute of Reconstructive Plastic Surgery at New York University Medical Center, Forward Face offers quarterly support meetings open to the public and a newsletter. (See Films and Videos section for Face Facts videotapes.) For more information, write: Patricia Chibbaro, RN, Institute of Reconstructive Surgery, H-148, 560 1st Ave, New York, NY 10016; or call (212) 263-5205.

Foundation for the Faces of Children

Contributions to the foundation support the Craniofacial Center of Children's Hospital Medical Center, Boston, in such areas as clinical, basic, and psychosocial research, postgraduate training in craniofacial surgery, and parent-to-parent support. Contributors receive a newsletter. For parent resource information or to address concerns, write to parent consultant Priscilla Bradway, PO Box 505, Weston, MA 02193; or call (508) 475-1077.

Happy Faces Support Group

Happy Faces provides education and support for people with facial differences and their families. Aside from local group meetings, Happy Faces will also make family visits upon request. For more information, contact Jaque Reiff, a craniofacial nurse specialist, at: 1331 N Seventh St, Ste 250, Phoenix, AZ 85006; or call (602) 252-3223.

Hemifacial Microsomia Family Support Network: Goldenhar Syndrome

This network offers support and education for parents and families of children born with hemifacial microsomia, including a free printout that describes hemifacial microsomia in lay terms and a newsletter. For more information, write: Cynthia and Richard Fishman, 6 Country Way, Philadelphia, PA 19115; or call (215) 677-4787. You may also write to Kayci Rush-Hall, a parent of a child with Goldenhar Syndrome, at: 3036 37th Ave S, Minneapolis, MN 55406; or call (612) 721-4590.

Let's Face It

An information and support network for people with facial differences, their families, friends, and professionals, Let's Face It, of Concord, Massachusetts, is the US branch of an international information and support network. Founded by Christine Piff, an Englishwoman who lost her palate and eye to cancer, Let's Face It is independent of any other support network. One of it's goals is to let people know they are not alone. The group handles calls from across the country and is able to link people to additional resources and networks. For additional information, write: Box 711, Concord, MA 01742-0004.

National Center for Education in Maternal and Child Health (NCEMCH) and National Maternal and Child Health Clearinghouse (NMCHC)

These sister organizations provide education and information services in maternal and child health. The center, NCEMCH, makes relevant information available through their many publications; a free catalog lists the materials according to specific topics. For more information write: NCEMCH/NMCHC, 2000 15th St, N, Ste 701, Arlington, VA 22201; or call NCEMCH (703) 524-7802; NMCHC (703) 821-8955 ext 254.

National Center for Youth with Disabilities

The center's mission is to improve the health and social functioning of youth with disabilities through technical assistance and consultation, dissemination of information, and increased coordination of services between the health-care system and other services. The Winter 1992 issue of *Connections*, the center's newsletter, discusses teen weight-control programs, sexual abuse of teens with disabilities, sexuality education program guidelines, and public attitudes toward people with disabilities. The center also offers training materials, new books, information on upcoming conferences, and youth trips. Write: NCYD Connections, University of Minnesota, Box 721 UMHC, Harvard St at E River Rd, Minneapolis, MN 55455; or call 1-800-333-6293 or (612) 626-2825.

National Foundation for Facial Reconstruction

The NFFR sponsors programs of the New York University Medical Center. A library of books and films is available to the public. For complete information, write: Arlyn Gardner, 317 E 34th St, 9th Floor, New York, NY 10016; or call (212) 263-6656; 1-800-422-FACE.

National Information Center for Children and Youth with Disabilities

The center, formerly called the National Information Center for Handicapped Children and Youth, is an information service that assists parents, educators, caregivers, and others in ensuring that all children and youths with disabilities have the opportunity to reach their potential. The center specializes in educational planning, but it also has information on a broad range of topics concerning the needs of children with handicaps. Material is available in large print or braille or can be taped upon request. The free newsletter includes a network exchange that allows people to share their experiences. Write: The National Information Center for Children and Youth with Disabilities, PO Box 1492, Washington, DC 20013; or call (703) 893-8614 (voice or TDD); or toll-free, 1-800-999-5599.

National Information System and Clearinghouse

The Clearinghouse, sponsored by the National Maternal and Child Health Bureau, offers information about children from birth to three years who have disabilities or life-threatening conditions and helps find services for children with special health-care needs or developmental disabilities. Parents and professionals are encouraged to use the center's free hotline and its resources. For more information, write: Center for Developmental Disabilities, University of South Carolina, Benson Bldg, First Floor, Columbia, SC 29208; or call (803) 777-4435; or toll-free 1-800-922-9234.

National Neurofibromatosis Foundation

With support groups located throughout the US, as well as a national newsletter, this foundation supports research and education for parents, patients, and professionals. For more information, write: National Neurofibromatosis Foundation, 141 Fifth Ave, Ste 7-S, New York, NY 10010; or call (212) 460-8980; toll-free 1-800-323-7938.

National Organization for Rare Disorders

NORD is an educational link for organizations and individuals concerned with rare disorders. It tracks legislation, researches diseases, advocates for funding, and awards grant money. *The Orphan Disease Update,* included with the $25 membership fee, addresses rare disorders and is mailed throughout the world. Annual meeting. For more information, write: NORD, PO Box 8923, New Fairfield, CT 06812-1783; or call (203) 746-6518.

Neurofibromatosis, Inc, Midatlantic Chapter

This organization for families and individuals offers free information about this neurologic genetic disorder, identifies local support groups, provides referrals to local medical resources, encourages research, and educates legislators about NF family needs. Newsletter; conferences. For more information, write: Mary Ann Wilson, 3401 Woodridge Ct, Mitchelville, MD 20721-2817; or call (301) 577-8984.

Prescription Parents, Inc

This active support network in New England for people with cleft lip and cleft palate offers outreach services to parents of newborns with cleft lip or palate. It also provides legislative advocacy, a newsletter, and social activities. For more information, write: Laura Cohen, PO Box 161, West Roxbury, MA 02132; or call (617) 527-0878.

Treacher Collins Foundation

Directed by a social worker and psychologist who have a child with Treacher Collins Syndrome, this foundation's primary goal is to link, through the TC Network, families and individuals affected by TC with each other and with professionals in the field of craniofacial anomalies in order to facilitate the development and sharing of their knowledge and experience. Newsletters; referral lists. For more information, write: Hope Charkins-Drazin and David Drazin, PO Box 683, Norwich, VT 05055; or call (802) 649-3020.

University of Connecticut Craniofacial Family Support Group

Serving over six hundred families in the Connecticut area with information, support, and meetings, this support group holds bimonthly conferences. Topics have included "Dealing with the Emotional Aspects of a Craniofacial Disorder" and "The Hows and Whys of Craniofacial Birth Defects." For more information, write: Rita Brzozowski, parent coordinator, University of Connecticut Craniofacial Family Support Group, 190 Tomlinson Ave, 12D, Plainville, CT 06062; or call (203) 793-1065.

Reading for Parents and Children

ACCH Parent Resource Directory

This paperback book contains a national list of parents who are available to talk with other parents who have a child with a similar disability. $5.00. To order, write: Association for the Care of Children's Health, 7910 Woodmont Ave, Ste 300, Bethesda, MD 20814; or call (301) 654-6549.

Advice to Parents of a Cleft Palate Child
D. Wicha and M. Folk

(2nd Ed; 1981), $12.25. To order, write: Charles C Thomas Publishing, 2600 S First St, Springfield, IL 62794-9265; or call (217) 789-8980.

Beauty Is the Beast
Ann Hill Beuf

Subtitled *Appearance-Impaired Children in America*, this book uses theory and methodology from sociology, anthropology, and psychology, as well as the author's interviews with children and their caretakers. Ms Beuf analyzes both the effects of stigmatization on children and the strategies used to cope. This book can be particularly meaningful for adults with facial disfigurement. 1990, $14.95. To order, call: University of Pennsylvania Press, (215) 898-6264.

Between Parent & Child
Between Parent & Teenager
Haim Ginott

Written by a children's psychiatrist, these books offer a means of building a loving dialogue with children and teenagers. The books have helped bring many parents and children together. Avon Books, 1969. Available through bookstores.

Brothers and Sisters: A Special Part of Exceptional Families
Thomas Powell and Peggy Ogle

Brothers and sisters of handicapped children are the focus of this book, which addresses such issues as the intensity of sibling relationships, sibling interactions, the factors contributing to a family's adjustment patterns, parental expectations, siblings as teachers, and siblings at school. Information and resources for siblings and parents are listed. 219 pp, paperback. To order, write: Paul H. Brookes Publishing Co, PO Box 10624, Baltimore, MD 21204.

Building the Healing Partnership: Professionals, and Children with Chronic Illness and Disabilities
Patricia Taner Leff, MD, and Elaine H. Walize

There are few crises as devastating as finding out that one's child is disabled or seriously ill—one of the themes of this powerful book designed for parents and health professionals. The authors, a psychiatrist and a mother of a special-needs child, cover all the implications of living with mental and physical disabilities. Having a "special" child puts the entire family at risk, and such families must perform extraordinary tasks day after day. The authors pull no punches; the talk is frank, alternately depressing and uplifting. Dozens of entries from parents and health-care workers aim to educate, invite change, and stimulate personal growth. A list of parent resources and a glossary are included. This book is excellent for parents, doctors, nurses, therapists, and teachers. Public and school libraries should consider ordering. (Book review by Linda Beck, Indian Valley Public Library, Telford, PA *[Library Journal]*). 1992, paperback, $24.95. To order, write: Brookline Books, Box 1046, Cambridge, MA 02238; or call (617) 868-0360 or (800) 666-2665.

A Button in Her Ear
Ada Litchfield

This book for children (ages 6–9) addresses the experiences of hearing-disabled children through the story of a girl with a hearing aid. To order, write: Albert Whitman Co, 6340 Oakton St, Morton Grove, IL 60053-2723; or call (708) 581-0033 or 1-800-255- 7675.

The Exceptional Parent

The Exceptional Parent is published eight times each year for parents of disabled children. Articles are written by parents of special-needs children, health-care and legal professionals, and individuals with disabilities. The "Reader's Forum" includes letters seeking and sharing information on treatment, supplies, services, and family experiences. Subscriptions: $18 per year for an individual, and $24 per year for an organization, library, school, or agency. Write: The Exceptional Parent, 1170 Commonwealth Ave, Third Floor, Boston, MA 02134-4646; or call (617) 730-5800.

Family Centered Care for Children with Special Health Care Needs
T. Shelton, E. Jeppson, and B. Johnson

This directory, affectionately known as "Big Red," is a wealth of resources for parents and professionals caring for children with chronic illness or disabling conditions. It discusses and lists family-centered care resources, including technical assistance, books, financial considerations, national programs and associations, references, and support groups. 74 pp. $8.50. To order, write: The Association for the Care of Children's Health, 7910 Woodmont Ave, Ste 300, Bethesda, MD 20814; or call (301) 654-6549.

How Different Is Anthony?
Joanne Green

Anthony was born with a cleft lip and palate, but does that really make him very different from other kids? This book helps children born with clefts to recognize themselves as the normal healthy kids they are. This is a self-esteem builder, designed to read aloud. Good for children of all ages, particularly those 4–8 years. To order, write: Wide Smiles/Anthony, PO Box 5753, Stockton, CA 95285- 8153.

Koko Bear's Big Earache (Preparing Your Child for Ear Tube Surgery)
V. Lansky

$5.95. (Bantam Books: Toronto, New York, London)

Meeting the Challenge: A Training Program for Adolescents with Special Needs
Kathleen Kapp-Simon

Adolescents with special needs are the topic of this training manual and accompanying video that focus on the development of interpersonal skills, self-awareness, and coping strategies. The manual and video provide theory, training strategies, and a curriculum. Featured in the videotape are several adolescents, some of whom have facial disfigurement. The program can be implemented by psychologists, nurses, social workers, child life specialists, or other professionals. Book, $30.00; book and video, $125.00; additional books with video, $25.00. To order, write:

Kathleen Kapp-Simon, UIC Craniofacial Center, Box 6998, Chicago, IL 60680; or call (312) 996-7546.

A Parent-Child Cleft Palate Curriculum: Developing Speech and Language
Bonnie L. Brookshire, MA, Joan I. Lynch EdD, and Donna R. Fox, PhD

Three experimental speech-language pathologists help parents to help their child with a cleft palate to speak well. To order, write: CC Publications, Inc, PO Box 23699, Tigard, OR 97223.

A Parent's Guide to Cleft Lip and Palate
K. Muller, C. Starr, and S. Johnson

"Should be required reading for every new parent of a child with a cleft," says one parent. Chapters range from a basic explanation of the current theory of the cause of clefts, to surgical repair and social and psychological development. To order, write: University of Minnesota Press, 2037 University Ave, SE, Minneapolis, MN 55414.

Rosey . . . The Imperfect Angel
Sandra Lee Peckinpah

Rosey is a positive, uplifting tale for all the world's different children, their parents, their brothers and sisters, their classmates and teachers—for anyone who has ever felt a little different. It is a tale told with real love that holds the promise of a happy ending. 1991, 32 pp. Cloth, $20.00. To order, write: Dasan Productions, 4201 Hunt Club Ln, Westlake Village, CA; or call 1-800-348-4401 or (818) 597-8380. Also available through: AboutFace, 1002 Liberty Ln, Warrington PA 18976; 1-800-225-FACE or (215) 491-0602; or in Canada: 99 Crown Ln, 3rd Floor, Toronto, ON, Canada MSR 3P4; (416) 944-FACE.

Wide Smiles Newsletter

While its focus is cleft lip and palate, this quarterly newsletter would also be of interest to parents of children with other craniofacial anomalies. Contributing articles and sharing advice are encouraged. Past articles have featured new studies and technologies, success stories, questions from parents, comments from teenagers, and book reviews. Future articles will focus on new feeding devices for children with cleft lip and palate. Subscription cost: $18.00 per year. For more information, or to subscribe, write: Joanne Green, PO Box 5153, Stockton, CA 95205-0153; or call (209) 942-2812.

Fun and Games

Danny's Song
Going to Sleep
I Am, I Can, I Will
Josephine, the Short-Necked Giraffe
Family Communications, Inc

In these combination books and audiotapes, Fred Rogers talks and sings about individual strengths and weaknesses and encourages children to explore all that they are. Also available are outstanding and reasonably priced videos, games, and toys. Videotapes preview hospital visits, having an operation, and how to deal with anger, rejection, jealousy, and fear, including the fear of death. Helpful to hospital staff, schools, and families, these packages are produced with the sensitive, creative spirit of any Mister Rogers' production. Write for a catalog: Family Communications, Inc, 4802 Fifth Ave, Pittsburgh, PA 15213; or call (412) 687-2990.

In The Hospital
Pluggin' Away
Moose School Records

These audiotapes by Peter Alsop and Bill Harley offer songs and stories created to help deal with the deepest feelings about being ill or different. Booklets accompany the taped stories and songs. One song, "Let's Face It," from *In the Hospital* was written by Peter Alsop for children with facial difference. *Pluggin' Away* includes such songs as "No One's Normal," "If I Was in Charge," "High Standards," and "I Can if I Wanna." (*In the Hospital*, $17.50; *Pluggin' Away*, $12.50.) Check your local music stores or order directly from: Moose School Records, Box 960, Topanga, CA 90290; or call (213) 445-2318.

Films and Videos

Center for Craniofacial Anomalies

What Is Going to Happen to My Baby?

This tape is an explanation of cleft lip and palate and an overview of the treatment provided by various disciplines at different stages of development. Audience: Parents and all health professionals associated with treatment of cleft lip/palate. Winner of the American Society of Plastic and Reconstructive Surgery Scientific Exhibit Award (15 min).

Feeding Your Special Baby

This tape shows modified feeding techniques for the baby born with cleft lip/palate. Audience: Parents, nurses, medical students, residents, pediatricians, and speech pathologists. Winner of two national awards of outstanding achievement in the use of television for education in the health sciences: Health Science Communications Association; and American Journal of Nursing Companies, Educational Services Division (15 min; also available in Spanish).

Your Baby's Surgery

An explanation of what a cleft is, how it is repaired,

and what hospitalization and postoperative care entails for a baby born with a cleft are the main topics of this concise and informative videotape (13 min).

Being Understood

This tape offers an overview of speech therapy for toddlers and older children with cleft palate. Audience: Parents, speech and language professionals, associated health professionals, and students (13 min).

Pharyngeal Flap

In accessible terms, this tape offers an explanation of speech mechanisms, hypernasal speech, and how pharyngeal flap surgery corrects this problem. Audience: Parents, patients, and all health professionals associated with cleft lip/palate (13 min; also available in Spanish).

SOM: A Silent Disease

This tape explains why children with cleft palate are susceptible to ear disease, offers advice on what can be done to prevent or correct ear disease in its early stages, and describes myringotomy surgery. Audience: Parents, patients, and all health professionals associated with cleft lip/palate (22 min; also available in Spanish).

Put on a Happy Face

Included here are the reasons children with cleft lip and palate need special attention to maintain good dental health, and a program to achieve this goal. Audience: Parents and all health professionals associated with cleft lip/palate (10 min; also available in Spanish).

All of these videotapes are available from the CCA to rent or to purchase. Rental fee is $30.00 for a 10-day period. Purchase price is $95.00. (Rental fee is applicable toward purchase price.) Postage and handling fees are added at time of shipment. To order, write: Marcia Aduss, CCA, University of Illinois College of Medicine at Chicago, PO Box 6998, Room 476 CME, M/C 588, Chicago, IL 60680.

Face Facts

Every maternity medical facility should own a copy of Face Facts' excellent 25-minute videos. They are designed for parents and families to use in the first days after the birth of a child with cleft lip and palate, craniosynostosis, hemifacial microsomia, orbital hypertelorism, or Treacher Collins syndrome. Narrated by Cliff Robertson, each tape includes an overview of the disorders and features in-depth interviews with medical professionals, educators, family members, and patients. An extended segment highlights specific family concerns.

Prices: $80.00 for a set of five to professionals and nonmembers (or $20.00 for a single tape); $60.00 for Forward Face members (or $15.00 for a single tape). All profits are used to develop future educational materials concerning craniofacial disorders and their treatment. For more information, write: Patricia Chibbaro, RN, Forward Face, Institute of Reconstructive Plastic Surgery, NYU Medical Center, 560 1st Ave, New York, NY 10016; or call (212) 263-5205, or 1-800-422-FACE.

Cleft Lip and Palate—Feeding the Newborn
Heartstar Productions, Ltd

Developed in 1992 by the Hospital for Sick Children's cleft lip and palate program, this videotape presents the appropriate methods to feed an infant with a cleft lip and/or palate (18 min). The tape sells for $95.00, but it is possible to preview the video at a cost of $10.00 (applicable toward the purchase price). For further information, or to order, contact: Sylvia Schippke, Coordinator, Cleft Lip and Palate

Program, Hospital for Sick Children, 555 University Ave, Toronto, Ontario, Canada, M5G 1X8; or call (416) 813-7490.

Feeding Aids

To order cleft palate bottles, contact: Mead Johnson Consumer Affairs, (812) 429-6321. For cleft palate NUK nipples, contact: Gerber Consumer Information Service: 1-800-4-GERBER.

Selected Bibliography of Publications on Cleft Lip and Palate

No single pamphlet is appropriate in its entirety for any given child. Please consult with the professional people who are caring for your child for a better understanding of the written materials as they may apply to your child's specific needs.

Cleft Palate Foundation Publications

All fees quoted are for professional institutions and organizations ordering in bulk; all CPF publications are free to parents. To order, contact: The Cleft Palate Foundation, 1218 Grandview Ave, Pittsburgh, PA 15211; or call 1-800-24-CLEFT. (See Appendix A for more on the CPF.)

For Parents of Newborn Babies with Cleft Lip/Palate
    1980, 4 pp. (.20)

A Los Padres de los Bebes Recién Nacidos con Labio Leporino/Paladar Hendido (Spanish-language version)
    1988, 4 pp. (.20)

Feeding an Infant with a Cleft
    1992, 11 pp. $1.75.

Cleft Lip and Cleft Palate: The First Four Years
    1989, 24 pp. $1.75.

Labio Henido y Paladar Hendido, los Cuatro Primeros Anos (Spanish language version)
    1989, 18 pp. $1.75.

Cleft Lip and Cleft Palate: The Child from Three to Twelve Years
    1980, 16 pp. $1.75.

Information for the Teenager Born with a Cleft Lip and/or Palate
    1980, 11 pp. $1.75.

The Genetics of Cleft Lip and Palate: Information for Families
    1987, 6 pp. $1.75.

Free Information from the Cleft Palate Foundation

Topics covered in these free pamphlets include:

Cleft Lip and Palate
Choosing a Cleft Palate or Craniofacial Team
Dental Care of a Child with Cleft Lip and Palate
Crouzon Syndrome (Craniofacial Dysostosis)
Pierre Robin Sequence
Treacher Collins Syndrome
Submucous Cleft Palate
Treatment for Adults with Cleft Lip and Palate
The National Cleft Palate Association
Financial Assistance

AboutFace Publications

(See Appendix C for more on AboutFace)

AboutFace
   General pamphlet. First copy free; multiple copies, .20 each.

Our Newborn Has a Facial Disfigurement
   Pamphlet. First copy free; multiple copies, .20 each.

Your Child and the Craniofacial Team
   Pamphlet. First copy free; multiple copies, .20 each.

Apert, Crouzon, and Other Craniosynostosis Syndromes
   Booklet. $2.00 each.

Making the Difference: A Resource for Health Care Providers
   Booklet. $3.00 each.

We All Have Different Faces: A School Education Program
   $17.00.

Manual for AboutFace Chapter Leaders and Area Representatives
   No charge for those interested in AboutFace chapter development.

Adoption Publications

Ours

For a one-year AFA membership fee of $24.00 you will receive this bimonthly magazine. It is also available in single copies for a $4.00 fee. To order, write: Adoptive Families of America, Inc, 3333 Highway 100 N, Minneapolis, MN 55422; or call (612) 535-4829.

Promising Smiles: Adopting a Child with Cleft Lip and Palate

This booklet was written to help prospective parents and waiting families with pre- and post-adoption tips and information. The format is one of parent-to-parent sharing. Discussion includes initial surgical procedures, treatment, feeding techniques, health insurance, professional services, special considerations in planning care, and suggestions to encourage speech and language development. Cost: approximately $5.00. Write: Friends of Love the Children, 21 S Auten Ave, Somerville, NJ 08876.

Hi Families

For a donation of $20.00 per year, you will receive this bimonthly newsletter in a color magazine format. Write: Holt Int'l Children's Services, PO Box 2880, Eugene, OR 97402.

Roots and Wings

For a $20.00 yearly fee, you will receive this quarterly publication with over 40 pages of adoption information, articles, stories, and photographs per issue. For a single copy there is a $5.00 fee. Write: NJ Friends Through Adoption, 161 Twin Brooks Tr, Chester, NJ 07930.

F.A.C.E. Facts

For a $20.00 yearly fee, you will receive this thick bimonthly newsletter with many stories of interest to adopting parents. Write: Families Adopting Children Everywhere, PO Box 28058, Northwood Station, Baltimore, MD 21239.

FAIR

For a $15.00 yearly fee, you will receive this thick bimonthly newsletter with a variety of interesting articles. Write: Families Adopting In Response, PO Box 51436, Palo Alto, CA 94303.

Other Publications and Books

Bright Promises
E. McDonald
 21 pp. $2.40. To order, contact: The National Easter Seal Society, 70 E Lake St, Chicago, IL 60601. (Also available in Spanish: *Un Futuro Prometedor: Para Su Niño Con Labio Hendido y Paladar Hendido)*

Cleft Lip and/or Palate: Will It Affect My Child
P. Starr
 1978, 43 pp. $1.00. To order, write: Lancaster Cleft Palate Clinic, 223 N Lime St, Lancaster, PA 17602.

Our Child with a Cleft Lip and Palate
L. Elms, A. Minerva, and P. Starr
 1978, 9 pp. $1.00. To order write: Lancaster Cleft Palate Clinic, 223 N Lime St, Lancaster, PA 17602.

Perspectives Concerning Cleft Lip and Cleft Palate
 1977, 91 pp. $4.50. Order through: Prescription Parents, Inc, PO Box 855, Quincy, MA 02169; or call (617) 479-2463.

The Child with Cleft Lip or Palate
M. Georgiade, E. Clifford, and R. Massengill
 21 pp. Free. Available through: The National Foundation/March of Dimes, Box 2000, White Plains, NY 10602.

Your Cleft Lip and Palate Child: A Basic Guide for Parents
G. Snyder, S. Berkowitz, K. Bzoch, and S. Stool
 1986, 14 pp. Free. Available through: Mead Johnson & Co, Nutritional Division, Evansville, IN 47721-0001.

Cleft Lip and Cleft Palate: Nursing Education Aids #11
 1962, 25 pp. Free. Available through: Ross Laboratories, 625 Cleveland Ave, Columbus, OH 43215.

Expressing Breast Milk: Hand Expression, Hand Pumping, Electric Pumping, Breast Milk Storage
S.C. Danner

1984. To order, write: Childbirth Graphics, Ltd, 2975 Brighton-Henrietta Townline Rd, Rochester, NY 14623.

Feeding Young Children with Cleft Lip and Palate
V. Bennett

$1.50. Available through: The Minnesota Dietetic Association, 1821 University Ave, W, Ste S-280, St Paul, MN 55104.

Nursing Your Baby with a Cleft Palate or Cleft Lip
S.C. Danner and E.R. Cerutti

1984. To order, write: Childbirth Graphics, Ltd, 2975 Brighton-Henrietta Townline Rd, Rochester, NY 14623.

Hearing and Behavior in Children Born with Cleft Palate

Booklet. To order, write: Prescription Parents, Inc, PO Box 855, Quincy MA 02169; or call (617) 479-2463.

Steps in Habilitation for the Cleft Lip and Palate Child
S. Berkowitz

13 pp, 1971. Free. Available through: Mead Johnson & Co, Evansville, IN 47721-0001.

The Road to Normalcy for the Cleft Palate Child
S. Berkowitz

1981, 13 pp. Free. Available through: Mead Johnson & Co, Evansville, IN 47721-0001.

Treatment of Deformities of the Face and Skull

Booklet. Published by the Tennessee Craniofacial Center. To order, write: Terri Farmer, Administrative Coordinator, Erlanger Medical Center, 975 E Third St, Chattanooga, TN 37403; or call 1-800-825-7002, or (615) 778-9191.

Howie Helps Himself

This story, for children ages 5–8, addresses the concerns of a boy with cerebral palsy. To order, write: Albert Whitman Co, 6340 Oakton St, Morton Grove, IL 60053-2723; or call (708) 581-0033 or 1-800-255-7675.

I'm Deaf and It's O.K.

This book, for children ages 6–9, offers an upbeat, realistic depiction of a young boy learning to accept his disability. To order, write: Albert Whitman Co, 6340 Oakton St, Morton Grove, IL 60053-2723; or call (708) 581-0033 or 1-800-255-7675.

Where's Chimpy?

This book, for children ages 3–7, explores the particular experience of a child with Down's Syndrome. To order, write: Albert Whitman Co, 6340 Oakton St, Morton Grove, IL 60053-2723; or call (708) 581-0033 or 1-800-255-7675.

Professional Textbooks

Plastic Surgery of the Facial Skeleton
S.A. Wolfe and S. Berkowitz
 Little, Brown: Boston, 1989

Communicative Disorders Related to Cleft Lip and Palate
K.B. Bzoch, ed
 College Hill (Little, Brown): Boston, 1989

The Cleft Palate Experience: New Perspectives on Management
E. Clifford
 Charles C Thomas: Springfield, IL, 1987

Cleft Palate Speech
B.J. McWilliams, H.L. Morris, and R.L. Shelton
   B.C. Decker: Philadelphia; and C.V. Mosby: St Louis, 1984

Developmental Craniofacial Biology
H.C. Slavkin
   Lea and Febiger: Philadelphia, 1979

Cleft Palate and Cleft Lip: A Team Approach to Clinical Management and Rehabilitation of the Patient
H.K. Cooper, R.L. Handing, W.M. Krogman, M. Mazaheri, and R.T. Millard
   W.B. Saunders: Philadelphia, 1979

Cleft Craft: The Evolution of Its Surgery, 3 vols
D.R. Millard, Jr.
   Little, Brown: Boston, 1977

Oral Facial Genetics
R.E. Stewart and G.H. Prescott
   C.V. Mosby: St Louis, 1976

Cleft Lip and Palate
R.B. Ross and M.S. Johnston
   Williams & Wilkins: Baltimore, 1972

Cleft Lip and Palate: Surgical, Dental, and Speech Aspects
W.C. Grabb, S.W. Rosenstein, and K.R. Bzoch, eds
   Little, Brown: Boston, 1971

Syndromes of the Head and Neck
R.J. Gorlin and J.J. Pindborg
   McGraw Hill: New York, 1964

Plastic Surgery, vol 4: Cleft Lip & Palate and Craniofacial Anomalies
Joseph G. McCarthy, MD, ed
   W.B. Saunders: Philadelphia, 1990

Craniosynostosis: Diagnostic Evaluation and Management
M. Michael Cohen, Jr, DMD, PhD, ed
Raven Press: New York, 1986

Craniofacial Surgery
Ernesto P. Caronne, MD, ed
Little, Brown: Boston, 1985.

Aesthetic Contouring of the Craniofacial Skeleton
Douglas K. Ousterhout, DDS, MD, ed
Little, Brown: Boston, 1991

Multidisciplinary Management of Cleft Lip and Palate
Janusz Bardach, MD, and Hughlett L. Morris, PhD, eds
W.B. Saunders: Philadelphia, 1990

Principlization of Plastic Surgery
D. Ralph Millard, Jr, MD
Little, Brown: Boston, 1986

Cleft Palate: Interdisciplinary Issues and Treatment—for Clinicians, by Clinicians
Karlind T. Moller, PhD and Clark D. Starr, PhD
Austin, TX: Pro-ed, 1993

Glossary

Allergic rhinitis   Swelling of the membrane in the nasal chamber due to allergic reactions; the condition may obstruct breathing

Alveolar ridge   The bony arches of the maxilla (upper jaw) and mandible (lower jaw) that contain the teeth

Alveolus   The bony area that supports the teeth

Anomaly   Irregularity

Anterior   Front

Appliance, dental   A device worn in the mouth to provide a dental benefit

Articulation   The process of forming and expressing speech sounds

Articulation disorder   The omission or ineffective expression of speech sounds

Articulation test   A test that evaluates how an individual's speech sounds are formed

Atelectasis   Collapse of eardrum, which separates the outer ear from the middle ear chamber

Atresia   The lack of closure of a normal body orifice or passage

Audiogram   A standard graph that records the results of hearing sensitivity testing

Audiologic evaluation   A variety of procedures used to measure hearing sensitivity

Audiologist   A person holding a degree and certification in audiology (the science of hearing), who identifies, measures, and rehabilitates people with hearing impairments

Audiology   The study of hearing and hearing disorders

Audiometer   An electronic instrument designed to measure hearing sensitivity

Bifid uvula   Uvula muscle divided into two parts

Bilateral   Having two sides, or pertaining to both sides

Bone graft   A transplant or movement of bone from one site to another

Braces   Orthodontic appliance attached to the teeth used to move them into a better position

Bridge   Fixed or removable appliance used to replace missing teeth and to help maintain the corrected dental arch form

Buccal   Pertaining to the cheek

Buccal segments of maxilla   The side portions of the upper jaw that are adjacent to the cheeks

Cephalometric tracing   Anatomic drawings made from x-ray films of the head

Cephalometric analysis   Head measurements made from the anatomic drawings of the head

Cineradiography   Motion picture recording of the lip, tongue, soft palate, and lower jaw activity; it is often used to evaluate the anatomic movements involved in speech

Cleft   Split or divided; refers to muscle, skin, or bone

Bilateral cleft: affecting both sides

Unilateral cleft: affecting only one side

Cleft lip   Congenital deformity of the upper lip that varies from a notching to a complete division of the lip; any degree of clefting can exist

Cleft palate   Split in the middle of the palate that may extend through the uvula, soft palate, and into the hard palate; the lip may or may not be involved in the cleft

Cleft palate craniofacial team Group of professionals involved in the care and treatment of patients having cleft palate and other craniofacial malformations; consists of representatives from some of the following specialties: pediatrics, plastic surgery, otolaryngology, audiology, speech pathology, pedodontics, psychiatry, orthodontics, prosthodontics, psychology, social service, nursing, radiology, genetics, and oral surgery

Columella The central lower portion of the nose that divides the nostrils

Communication disorder Any interference with one's ability to comprehend or express ideas, experiences, knowledge, and feelings

Comprehension Knowledge or understanding of spoken and written information

Congenital A disease, deformity, or deficiency existing at birth

Craniofacial Involving the cranium, or part of the skull that encloses the brain, and the face

Crossbite occlusion Condition in which the upper teeth are positioned behind the lower teeth, instead of in the normal position

Deciduous teeth The first teeth, known as baby or primary teeth, which are eventually replaced by permanent teeth

Denasality A lack of nasal quality of the voice; there is a lack of nasal resonance for the sounds *m*, *n*, and *ng* due to insufficient nasal air flow

Dental arch The curved structure of the upper and lower jaws formed by the teeth in their normal position on the alveolar ridges

Dental crown Cover for a tooth that is made by a dentist

Ear The organ of hearing, which is divided into three parts: the outer, middle, and inner ear

Ear canal The external canal leading from the outer ear to the eardrum (tympanic membrane)

Eardrum Tympanic membrane; it vibrates and transmits sound from the canal to the middle ear

Effusion Accumulation of fluid in the middle ear

E.N.T. Common medical abbreviation for "ear, nose, and throat"

Erupt, eruption The emergence of a tooth through the gums and its supporting bone

Eustachian tube The air duct that connects the nasopharynx (located in the back of the throat and above the hard [bony] palate) with the middle ear; it is usually closed at one end, but opens with yawning and swallowing; it allows ventilation of the middle ear cavity and equalization of pressure on both sides of the eardrum

Evaluation Assessment

Expander Appliance used to widen the upper dental arch

Extraction Removal (in this case, of teeth)

Fistula Abnormal opening from the mouth to the nasal cavity remaining after surgical closure of the original cleft

Genetics The science of heredity

Gingiva Gums

Hard palate The bony portion of the roof of the mouth

"Hare lip" Outdated term for cleft lip

Hearing impairment A loss in hearing, ranging from mild to complete

Heredity Characteristics and traits genetically derived from one's ancestors

Hypernasality Excessive nasal resonance during speech due to an excess of air flow into the nasal chamber

Hyponasality Lack of nasal resonance during speech due to a marked decrease in air flow

Impedance audiometry Physiologic hearing test used to measure air pressure in the middle ear cavity and the ability of the eardrum to function normally

Incidence Frequency of occurrence

Incisor A tooth that is located in the front of the mouth between the cuspids

Inferior Lower

Inner ear The internal portion of the ear that contains the sensory end organs used for hearing and balance

Intermaxillary fixation The use of elastics and/or wires to stabilize the upper to lower arches after surgery to one or both jaws

Language disorder or impairment Difficulty with language comprehension or expression; an interference with the ability to communicate effectively

Larynx The upper part of the windpipe that contains the vocal chords

Lateral Relating to the side

Logan's bow An appliance used to keep the lips together before lip surgery to reduce tension at the suture site

Malocclusion A deviation from normal occlusion (the way the teeth should meet), or an incorrect alignment or position of the upper with the lower teeth; any number of teeth may be involved

Mandible U-shaped bone forming the lower jaw

Mandibular Relating to the mandible or lower jaw

Maxilla The bone forming the upper jaw

Maxillary Relating to the maxilla or upper jaw

Maxillary orthopedics The movement of palatal segments by the use of appliances

Medial In, near, or positioned toward the middle

Micrognathia A condition characterized by abnormal smallness of the jaw

Middle ear Portion of the ear containing the three small bones of the ossicular chain that transfers sound from the eardrum to the inner ear; it is attached to the tympanic membrane on one end and the oval window at the other end

Mucoperiosteum Connective tissue (periosteum) that has a mucous surface that contacts bone on one side

Mucosa The outer layer of the soft tissue lining that covers the bone (in this case, in the mouth)

Multifactorial Having many factors or causes

Myringotomy A minor surgical procedure in which a small slit is made in the eardrum, allowing fluid to drain from the middle ear; it may or may not involve placement of ventilating tubes

Nasal   Pertaining to the nose or nasal cavity

Nasal alae   The wings of the nostrils

Nasal cavity   Passageway from the nostrils to the back of the throat

Nasal chamber   The enclosed space within the nose

Nasal emission or nasal escape   The flow of air through the nose, usually indicative of an incomplete seal between the cavities of the mouth and the nose

Nasopharyngoscope   A lighted telescopic instrument used for examining the nasal passages in the back of the throat; it is also useful in assessing velopharyngeal closure

Nasopharynx   The area in the back of the throat, at and above the soft palate

Obturator   A plastic (acrylic) appliance, usually removable, used to close a cleft in the hard palate; it is sometimes used to aid in feeding

Occlude   To block

Occlusion   Relationship between the upper and lower teeth when they are in contact; it refers to the alignment of teeth as well as the relationship of the dental arches

Oral cavity   The mouth, whose boundaries are the lips and teeth in the front and the soft palate in the rear

Orofacial   Relating to the mouth and face

Oropharynx   The area of the pharynx below the soft palate and above the esophagus and continuous with the mouth

Orthodontics   The specialty of dentistry concerned with the correction and prevention of irregularities and malocclusion of the teeth and jaws

Orthognathic   Dealing with the cause and treatment of malposition of the jaw bones

Orthopedics   The movement of bone by means of appliances rather than surgery

Ossicles   Three bones in the middle ear that transfer energy from sound waves in the tympanic membrane into the inner ear, where hearing sensors are located

Otitis media   Inflammation of the middle ear, where thick mucous fluid accumulates; this is a special problem for infants with cleft palates

Otolaryngologist Physician specializing in the diagnosis and treatment of diseases of the ear and larynx; commonly referred to as an ear, nose, and throat (E.N.T.) specialist

Otoscope An instrument used for visual examination of the external ear and eardrum

Overbite The distance of the upper to lower teeth in the vertical dimension

Overjet The distance between the upper and lower teeth in the horizontal dimension

Palatal insufficiency Velopharyngeal insufficiency; the inability to control air flow through the nose and mouth (too much air enters the nose)

Palatal lift appliance A removable plastic appliance with an extension reaching backward that lifts the soft palate

Palate The roof of the mouth, including the front portion or hard palate, and the rear portion or soft palate (velum)

Pediatrician Physician specializing in pediatrics, the area of medicine dealing with the health and diseases of children and adolescents

Pediatric dentist A dentist specializing in dental care for children and adolescents

Pedodontics Pediatric dentistry: the specialty of dentistry concerned with the care of children's and adolescent's teeth

Periosteum Connective tissue layer that covers bones

Pharyngeal Relating to the pharynx, the back of the throat

Pharyngeal flap A surgical procedure that aids in velopharyngeal closure; a flap of skin (mucosa) taken from the back of the throat and attached to the soft palate is used to close most of the openings between the oropharynx and nasopharynx during swallowing and speech

Pharynx Back of the throat

Posterior Back

Premaxilla The front part of the upper jaw containing the front teeth (the incisors); in children with clefts to the alveolus the number of incisor teeth is highly variable

Prolabium   The central part of the lip attached to the premaxilla

Prosthesis   A device used to replace a missing body part, in this case teeth to maintain the upper jaw arch form and/or to aid speech function

Retrognathic   Lower or upper jaw behind its normal position as related to the opposing jaw and other craniofacial structures

Rigid fixation   The use of metal plates and/or screws to stabilize bone manipulated by surgery

Septum, nasal   Dividing wall or partition between the two nasal cavities

Simonart's band   Bands of soft tissue (skin and muscle) that bridge a cleft of the lip

Sphincter pharyngoplasty   A surgical procedure used to channel the flow of air through the mouth by reducing the nasopharyngeal opening

Superior   Upper

Teratogen   Something causing physical defects in the developing embryo

Tympanic membrane   Eardrum

Unilateral   One-sided

Uvula   Muscle extension on the soft palate that can be seen as fleshy lobe in the midline of the throat; it is thought to aid in air-flow control

Velopharyngeal   Pertaining to the soft palate and pharynx

Velopharyngeal incompetence   Inadequate velopharyngeal closure resulting in hypernasality (excessive flow of air through the nose); also called Velopharyngeal insufficiency

Velum   The soft palate

Vomer (adj., vomerine)   The bony part of the nasal partition that separates the nose into right and left halves; it is attached to the hard palate

*I*ndex

Pages with illustrations or text and illustrations are indicated in italics.